MW01489354

DERMATOLOGY

Edited by
Kimberly N. Jones, M.D.
Barbara B. Wilson, M.D.

WYSTERIA
Long Island, New York
www.wysteria.com

Library of Congress Cataloging-in-Publication Data

Jones, Kimberly N.
    Dermatology / Kimberly N. Jones, Barbara B. Wilson.
        p.; cm.-- (Pocket brain)
    Includes bibliographical references.
    ISBN 0-9677839-6-8
    1. Skin--Diseases--Handbooks, manuals, etc. 2. Dermatology--Handbooks, manuals, etc.
I. Wilson, Barbara B. II. Title. III. Series.
    [DNLM: 1. Skin Diseases--Handbooks.   WR 39 J77d2002]
RL74.J66 2002
616.5--dc21

                                                        2002016805

Printed in the U.S.A.
ISBN 0-9677839-6-8

CONTENTS

1

APPROACH TO THE DERMATOLOGIC PATIENT

Dermatological lesions may be the symptomatic result of a primary skin process or a manifestation of a systemic illness. The etiologies include infectious, hereditary, auto-immune, traumatic, neoplastic, allergic, toxic, vascular, endocrine, environmental, psychological, response to sun exposure, and many others.

Epidemiology
   Age
   Race
   Sex
   Occupation

HPI
   Duration
   Cold/Hot
   Hobbies
   Menses
   Pets
   Pregnancy
   Season
   Travel

Medications/Allergies

Family History
   History of skin cancer or other relevant information

Symptoms
   Pruritus
   Pain
   Paresthesia
   Photosensitivity

Constitutional symptoms
   Acute: Headache, chills, fever, weakness
   Chronic: Fatigue, weakness, anorexia, weight loss

General Review of Systems

1

Physical Exam for the dermatologic patient: Carefully describe the lesion:

SIZE

  Flat

    Macule   < 0.5 cm

    Patch   > 0.5 cm

  Raised

    Papule   < 0.5 cm

    Nodule   > 0.5 cm in depth and diameter

    Tumor   synonymous with large nodule

  Raised with flat top

    Plaque   > 0.5 cm without significant depth

    Wheal   change rapidly, disappears in hours

  Fluid filled blister (clear)

    Vesicle   < 0.5 cm

    Bulla   > 0.5 cm

  Fluid filled (purulent exudate)

    Pustule

SURFACE

  Ulcer- skin defect characterized by loss of epidermis and papillary dermis.

  Scaly- psoriasis, solar keratosis, see papulosquamous.

  Crusts- impetigo, ecthyma.

EVOLUTION (stages of each lesion, and progression of pattern of all lesions).

SITE localized, diffuse, progression from proximal to distal or distal to proximal.

SHAPE of each lesion, of pattern of lesions together.

EDGE/BORDER sharp, irregular, elevated, etc.

COLOR

ODOR

TENDERNESS on palpation or spontaneously, or non-tender.

CONSISTENCY on palpation: hard, soft, etc.

LYMPHADENOPATHY local or distal.

OTHER SIMILAR LESIONS concurrently or in the past.

ALSO NOTE HAIR, NAILS, MUCOUS MEMBRANES

Special tests:

  DIASCOPY: press microscope slide or magnifying glass against lesion.

    Blanching- dilated capillaries (erythema)

    Nonblanching- extravasated blood (purpura)

    Translucent yellow brown- granulomas

      seen in sarcoidosis, tuberculosis, lymphoma, necrobiosis lipoidica.

  KOH 2 drops of 10-20% on slide to dissolve keratin for fungal elements.

    Heating accelerates the process.

  TZANCK SMEAR To evaluate for multinucleated giant cells of Herpes virus,

    scrape the base of an early vesicle, air dry or fix with ethanol,

    stain with Giemsa or Wright's stain.

  WOOD'S LAMP

      Yellow to green- some Dermatophytes

      Coral red- Erythrasma

      Pale blue- Pseudomonas

      Dark pink urine- Porphyria

      Completely white- Vitiligo

SOME USEFUL DESCRIPTIVE TERMINOLOGY

Dermatologists have their own unique vocabulary to help differentiate one skin lesion from another. These terms are used to communicate size, shape, color, texture, discharge, surface characteristics, growth characteristics, geometric pattern formation, location related to skin layers or skin components, function of skin components, inflammatory response, response to diascopy, etc. The following terms are most useful for purely descriptive purposes.

Annular - ring shaped.

Arciform - bow shaped.

Atrophic- wasting away of tissue or organ.

Atopic- allergic.

Blancheable - pallor or loss of color upon compression.

Blister - vesicle or bulla occurring between epidermis and dermis or within dermis.

Bullae - fluid filled cystic structure > 0.5 cm.

Burrow -sinus or fistula furrowed into the skin by a parasite.

Cicatrix - scar.

Corium- dermis.

Crust - dried liquid debris (puss or serous fluid) that has been deposited on the surface of skin.

Cutis - skin.

Cyst - vesicle filled with liquid or semi-solid material, located between dermis and epidermis.

Erosion- lesion characterized by loss of the epidermis only, see ulcer.

Eruption - breakout of a rash on the skin.

Erythematous - redness of the skin due to hyperemia.

Eschar - dry scab.

Exantham - skin eruption caused by action of infectious microorganisms or their toxins on skin blood vessels.

Excoriation - breaking away of superficial layers of skin due to scratching or scrapping.

Exfoliation - skin peeling off in scales or sheets.

Fissure - a linear tear in epidermis.

Granuloma - tumor composed of granulation tissue.

Hypermelanosis - excessive deposits of melanin from melanocytes.

Hyperplasia - over growth of tissue due to increase in number of constituent cells.

Hypertrophic - over growth of tissue due to increased size of constituent cells.

Induration - the hardening and thickening of tissue.

Integument - skin.

Lichenified - characterized by a thickened epidermis.

Macule - discoloration of epidermis; not elevated.

Mole - any pigmented fleshy or papula growth of skin.

Nodule - large abnormal aggregation of cells in the epidermis (> 0.5 cm in breadth and depth).

Papilliform - resembling multiple papilla or multiple small nipple-like projections.

Papule - small abnormal aggregation of cells in the epidermis (< 0.5 cm in breadth and depth).

Patch - macule with some skin surface scaling or wrinkling.

Plaque - elevated lesion of superficial epidermis >0.5 cm breadth, without significant depth.

Pruritus- itchiness.

Punctate - highly circumscribed like a point.

Rhytides - wrinkles.

Scale - thickened stratum corneum that becomes white and dry and flakes off.

Scar - fibrous connective tissue replacement of mesodermal and ectodermal tissue that has been destroyed by injury or disease.

Stellate - shaped like a star.

Target - ring shaped or multiple concentric ring shaped lesions.

Ulcer- characterized by loss of the epidermis and papillary dermis, see erosion.

Vesicle - fluid filled cystic structure <0.5 cm.

Violaceous - characterized by a violet color.

Wheal (hive)- a pruritic pink to red polymorphous plaque occurring secondary to a cutaneous immune response, which is usually transient. See urticaria.

Wrinkle - loss of elastic recoil of skin usually due to a degeneration of elastin fibers but can also be due to over growth of elastin fibers.

3

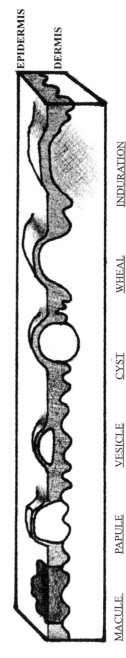

EPIDERMIS

DERMIS

MACULE
PATCH if
surface changes

PAPULE
NODULE if
larger than .5cm

VESICLE
BULLA if
larger than .5cm

CYST
PUSTULE if
filled with pus

WHEAL
Intradermal
inflammation

INDURATION
Dermal hardening
and thickening

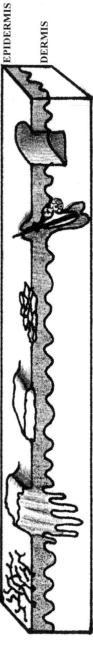

EPIDERMIS

DERMIS

TELANGIECTASIA

LICHENIFIED

PLAQUE
Larger than .5cm

SCALE
White and flaky

COMEDO
Hair follicle plug

ULCER
EROSION if only
epidermal depth

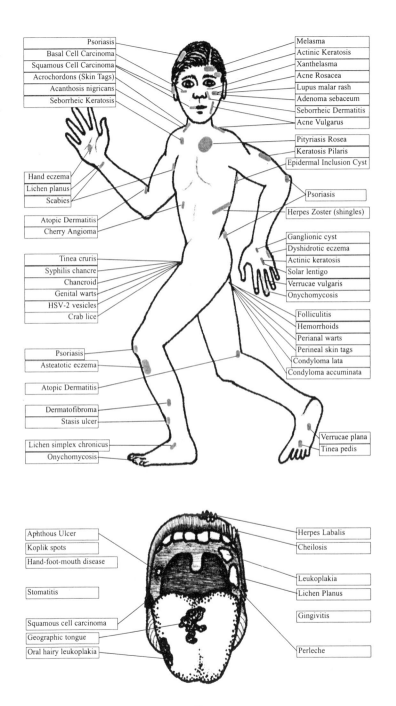

Psoriasis
Basal Cell Carcinoma
Squamous Cell Carcinoma
Acrochordons (Skin Tags)
Acanthosis nigricans
Seborrheic Keratosis

Melasma
Actinic Keratosis
Xanthelasma
Acne Rosacea
Lupus malar rash
Adenoma sebaceum
Seborrheic Dermatitis
Acne Vulgarus

Pityriasis Rosea
Keratosis Pilaris
Epidermal Inclusion Cyst

Hand eczema
Lichen planus
Scabies

Atopic Dermatitis
Cherry Angioma

Psoriasis

Herpes Zoster (shingles)

Tinea cruris
Syphilis chancre
Chancroid
Genital warts
HSV-2 vesicles
Crab lice

Ganglionic cyst
Dyshidrotic eczema
Actinic keratosis
Solar lentigo
Verrucae vulgaris
Onychomycosis

Folliculitis
Hemorrhoids
Perianal warts
Perineal skin tags
Condyloma lata
Condyloma accuminata

Psoriasis
Asteatotic eczema

Atopic Dermatitis

Dermatofibroma
Stasis ulcer

Lichen simplex chronicus
Onychomycosis

Verrucae plana
Tinea pedis

Aphthous Ulcer
Koplik spots
Hand-foot-mouth disease

Stomatitis

Squamous cell carcinoma
Geographic tongue
Oral hairy leukoplakia

Herpes Labialis
Cheilosis

Leukoplakia
Lichen Planus

Gingivitis

Perleche

5

2

SKIN HISTOLOGY AND PHYSIOLOGY

FUNCTIONS-

Mechanical and solar protection; multimodal sensation; thermoregulation.

LAYERS (outer to inner)

EPIDERMIS:-

Stratum corneum-

Flattened cell remnants without nuclei; contain intracytoplasmic keratin.

Stratum lucidum-

Thin region of homogenous material present in thick skin.

Stratum granulosum-

Contain keratohalin granules and tonofibrils; involved in keratinization.

Stratum spinosum-

Polyhedral cells attached via visible desmosomes. Site of active synthesis of cytokeratin.

Stratum basale-

Single layer of cuboidal cells attached to basement membrane by hemi-desmosomes. Melanocytes found here.

Basement membrane

DERMO-EPIDERMAL JUNCTION:- site of free sensory nerve endings.

DERMIS:-

Papillary dermis-

Fibroblasts interspersed among loosely arranged fine collagen and elastin fibrils. Contains papillary arterial loops, subpapillary vessel systems, axonal connections to free nerve endings in the epidermis, arrector pili, Meissner's corpuscles, mast cells hair shafts, and sebaceous glands.

Reticular dermis-

Fibroblasts interspersed in coarse collagen and elastin fibrils. Contains blood vessels connecting the subpapillary arterial system to the deeper cutaneous arterial plexus, hair follicles, sebaceous glands, sweat glands (both eccrine and apocrine), mast cells, and nailbeds.

HYPODERMIS:-

Loosely arranged adipose/areolar tissue. Contains base of hair follicles, base of sebaceous glands and sweat glands, and deep arterial/venous connections.

SKIN COMPONENTS:

Apocrine sweat glands- coiled exocrine glands with dilated lumens found in genital regions, nipples, and axilla; part of the secreting cell is cast off along with the secreted substance.

Arrector pili- smooth muscle bundle responsible for hair erection. Located in papillary dermis.

Eccrine (Merocrine) sweat glands- coiled exocrine glands with small lumen found dispersed over most of the body; secreting cell remains intact upon discharge of secreted substance.

Krause end bulbs- sensory nerve receptors found in conjunctiva and oropharynx.

Glomus bodies- dermal arterial-venous shunts located in distal sites (such as the external ear, toes, and fingertips) exposed to cool temperatures.

Langerhan's cells- antigen-presenting cells in the skin.

Mast cells- contain histamine, located in dermal connective tissue.

Meissner's corpuscles- small encapsulated sensory receptors scattered throughout the papillary dermis in fingerstips, genitalia, nipples, eyelids, and soles of feet. For light touch sensation.

Melanin- substance produced, secreted and distributed by melanocytes for skin pigmentation.

Melanocytes- melanin-producing cells of neuroectodermal origin found within the basal layers of the epidermis.

Merkel cells- non-neuronal cells associated with a terminal expansion of free sensory nerve endings within the papillary dermis.

Pacinian corpuscles- large encapsulated sensory receptors scattered throughout ligaments, joints, viscera, genitalia, and deep dermis of thick skin. Responsive to coarse mechanical stimuli - pressure.

Ruffini corpuscles- spindle shaped sensory receptors found in feet soles -pressure and warmth.

Sebum- oily substance secreted by sebaceous glands.

Sebaceous glands- produce sebum, secrete into hair follicle.

Sweat- perspiration: Eccrine sweat glands, superficial, produce liquid that contains water, sodium chloride, urea, albumin. Apocrine sweat glands, deep in axilla, produce similar liquid but with the addition of organic substances which react with local bacteria to produce and offensive odor.

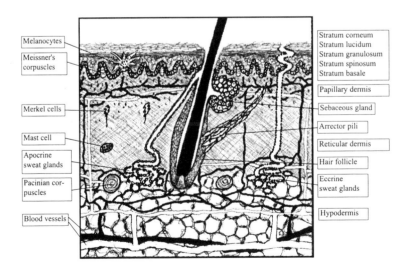

3

NEVI AND OTHER PIGMENTED LESIONS

BLUE NEVUS
Description- dark blue to black papule or nodule.
Pathology- benign proliferation of melanin-producing dermal melanocytes.
Rx- rarely malignant. Observe for changes.

BECKER'S NEVUS
Description- benign pigmented hamartoma on shoulder, characterized by
   hypertrichosis, usually occurring in teenage boys.
Pathology- increased melanin in basal keratinocytes; acanthosis; hyperkeratosis.
Rx- excise if a cosmetic concern, no increased risk of melanoma.

CAFE AU LAIT MACULES
Description- large tan to brown macules which may be found in high numbers
   in patients affected with Albrights's syndrome or neurofibromatosis.
Pathology- melanin macroglobules (more than 10 per 5 HPF).
Rx-benign

COMPOUND NEVUS
Description- tan to brown papule or nodule with uniform to mottled color.
Pathology- nests of melanocytes at the dermoepidermal junction and dermis.
Rx- observe for change. Compound nevi may evolve into intradermal nevi.
   Consider removal if on soles, mucous membranes, anogenital region, or scalp,
   if color variegated, border irregular, if lesion is symptomatic or if it is changing.

DERMATOFIBROMA
Definition- firm red, blue, brown nodule that dimples with lateral pressure.
   Common in lower extremities, may be related to minor trauma.
Pathology- increased pigmentation of epidermis, nodular aggregation of fibroblasts
   and densely packed collagen.
Rx-benign

DYSPLASTIC NEVUS
Description- brown to dark brown variegated moles with irregular borders;
   thought to be a marker of persons with increased risk for developing melanoma.

Pathology- increased number and size of spindle-shaped melanocytes, nuclear and cell body pleomorphism, reduced adhesiveness and bridging between rete ridges.
Rx- excise

EPHELIDES (freckles)
Description- hyperpigmented macules, darken upon sun-exposure.
Pathology- increased melanin in epidermis basal layer, no increase in melanocytes.
Rx- benign.

HALO NEVUS
Description- brown papule surrounded by round region of depigmentation. Occurs especially in patients with family history of or predilection for vitiligo.
Pathology- cytotoxic immune response against melanocytes.
Rx- reassure patient. Remove if mole demonstrates any worrisome features.

INTRADERMAL NEVUS
Description- flesh-colored or pigmented; soft papule or nodule; may be cerebriform or dome-shaped with terminal hairs.
Pathology- nests of melanocytes in the dermis.
Rx- observe for changes. In the final stage of evolution, it may become fibrotic. Remove if mole is bothersome or shows any worrisome changes.

JUNCTIONAL NEVUS
Description- brown to black macule with uniform color.
Pathology- nests of melanocytes at the dermoepidermal junction.
Rx- observe for changes. Consider removal if on soles, mucous membranes, anogenital region, or scalp, if color variegated, border irregular, if lesion is symptomatic or if it is changing.

LENTIGO SIMPLEX
Description- small oval to round tan, brown to black macule. Similar to freckles but do not darken with sun exposure.
Pathology- increased number of melanocytes not arranged in nests.

MELASMA
Description- regions of hyperpigmentation in sun-exposed areas, can be associated with hormonal modulation such as in pregnancy or use of oral contraceptives.
Pathology- increased production of melanosomes.
Rx- topical treinoin and hydroquinone solution (3%).

MELANOMA (see also Melanoma chapter)
Description- ABCD's: Asymmetry; Border irregularities; Color abnormalities (especially black, and numerous colors within one mole); Diameter greater than 6mm (a pencil eraser).
Pathology- malignant neoplastic transformation of melanocytes.
Stages- I: <1.5cm. II: >1.5cm. III: spread to lymph nodes. IV: distant metastases.
Rx- Surgical excision with wide margin, and regional lymph node dissection. Adjuvant therapy with chemotherapy, immunotherapy, and radiation therapy. Surgical resection of metastatic lesions (brain, viscera). Palliative care (incurable if metastatic).

9

MELANOMA SUB-TYPES:

Acral lentiginous melanoma- most common melanoma of Asian and African populations, dark brown, black, or bluish macule that occurs in mucocutaneous skin, genitalia, nail bed, sole, or palm regions; may be sub-ungual.
Pathology- nests of large spindle shaped melanocytes with dendrites, usually characterized by lymphocytic infiltration of the dermal-epidermal junction.

Desmoplastic melanoma- blue to gray macule, papule, or nodule lacks melanin and often occurs on face and neck.
Pathology- solitary or nests of atypical melanocytes located in the epidermis. Spindle-shaped cells interspersed between wide collagen fibrils located in the dermis, S-100 positive, occasionally HMB-45 negative.

Lentigo maligna melanoma- rarest of the 3 major types. characterized by a white to black variegated macule located on the face or arms.
Pathology- nest of melanocytes in basal epidermis, involves hair follicles early.

Nodular melanoma- sharply defined blue-black nodule, mostly in Japanese.
Pathology- large melanocytes primarily invading the epidermis and dermis in a vertical direction.

Superficial spreading melanoma- most common melanoma characterized by irregular borders, variegated color, and sharply demarcated elevated plaque.
Pathology- large melanocytes containing abundant cytoplasm spreading along the epidermis, usually S100 and HMB-45 positive.

NEVUS OF OTA
Description- non-heritable blue-brown mottled pigmentation of skin and mucous membranes. Characteristic of Asian, African, and East Indian populations. Nevus of Ota usually involves the distribution of the first and second branches of the trigeminal nerve; it may be disfiguring.
Pathology- ectopic dermal melanocytes produce a blue pigment.
Rx- pigmented lesion lasers.

NEVUS SPILUS (Nevus with spots)
Description- tan patch containing many smaller dark brown macules or papules.
Pathology- increased number of melanocytes with scattered junctional or compound nevi.
Rx- rarely contain dysplastic nevi. Observe for atypia and change.

SEBORRHEIC KERATOSIS
Description- verrucous, velvety, scaling, slow-growing, brown, grey, black, flesh-colored, or pink; macules/papules; sharply demarcated "stuck on" appearance. Other characteristics include plugged follicles (horn cysts) which is almost pathognomonic.
Pathology- keratinocyte and melanocyte proliferation.
Rx- electrocautery or cryosurgery. Specimen should be sent for histopathologic examination if diagnosis is in question.

SOLAR LENTIGO

Description- yellow to dark brown macules ranging in size from 10 to 30 mm, which result from a local proliferation of normal melanocytes in response to chronic sun exposure; but, unlike freckles, do not darken with sun exposure. Commonly occur on back of hand, and forehead of elderly light skin people. Also known as senile lentigo or liver spots.

Pathology- increased melanocytes and hypermelanosis, elongated rete ridges.

SPITZ NEVUS

Description- solitary or multiple pink to tan, often rapidly growing, dome-shaped papules occurring in children.

Pathology- epithelioid and spindle cells; sometimes difficult to distinguish histologically from melanoma.

Rx- excise.

4

DIFFERENTIAL DIAGNOSES

ACNEIFORM/PUSTULAR ERUPTIONS:
Acne vulgaris
Pityrosporum ovale/orbiculare folliculitis
Acne rosacea
Perioral dermatitis
Medications (please see medication reactions)
    Corticosteroids
    Other
Toxins
    Dioxin
    Herbicides
    Other chlorinated aromatic hydrocarbons
Systemic diseases
    Androgenic excess
    Polycystic ovary disease
    Cryptococcosis

ALOPECIA Nonscarring
Primary
    Alopecia areata
    Telogen effluvium
    Anagen effluvium
Cutaneous disease
    Eczema
    Local allergens/irritants
    Psoriasis
    Seborrheic dermatitis
Endocrinopathies
    Androgenic alopecia
    Hyperthyroidism (hair is also fine & soft)
    Hypothyroidism (hair is brittle, coarse, & dry)
Infectious
    Tinea capitis
    HIV
    Secondary syphilis

Medications (please see medication reactions)
Nutritional
    Anorexia nervosa/sudden weight loss
    Biotin deficiency
    Kwashiorkor
    Marasmus
    Iron deficiency
    Zinc deficiency
Psychiatric
    Trichotillomania
Systemic disease
    Connective tissue diseases
Stress (physical/emotional)
    Telogen effluvium

ALOPECIA Scarring
Idiopathic
    Pseudopelade of Brocq
    Dissecting cellulitis
    Acne keloidalis (more common in African men)
    Pseudofolliculitis barbae (more common in African men)
    Central centrifugal scarring alopecia
        Folliculitis decalvans
        Follicular degeneration syndrome
    Cicatricial pemphigoid
    Lichen planopilaris
    Morphea/scleroderma
    Sarcoidosis
    Aplasia cutis congenita
Infectious
    Bacterial (pyogenic infections)
    Fungal (kerion or blastomycosis)
    Viral (VZV, variola)
    Protozoal (leishmaniasis)
    Mycobacterial (leprosy, TB)
    Spirochetal (tertiary syphilis)
Neoplastic
    Basal cell carcinoma
    Squamous cell carcinoma
    Lymphoma
    Metastatic carcinoma
    Adnexal tumors
Physical
    Burn (fire, acid, alkali, curling iron, and radiation)
    Freeze
    Trauma (traction)
    Factitious

ANNULAR LESIONS (Target lesions)

<u>Primary cutaneous disease</u>
    Granuloma annulare
    Tinea corporis

<u>Systemic</u>
    Migratory
        Urticaria
        Erythema gyratum repens
        Erythema marginatum
        Erythema migrans
        Erythema annulare centrifugum
        Glucagonoma syndrome (Necrolytic migratory erythema)
    Nonmigratory
        Sarcoidosis
        Subacute cutaneous lupus erythematosus
        Secondary syphilis
        CTCL (Cutaneous T-cell Lymphoma)

CHEILITIS (Inflammation of the lips)
Accutane
Actinic
Contact dermatitis (mango peel, etc.)
Habitual lip-licking
Pellagra
Vitamin B12 deficiency

CONTACT DERMATITIS

<u>Irritant</u>
    Soap
    Cold weather
    Detergents
    Solvents
    Cements
    Cutting oils

<u>Allergic</u>
    Rhus dermatitis (poison oak, ivy, or sumac)
    Rubber (accelerators)
    Nickel
    Neomycin
    Paraphenylenediamine (hair dyes)
    Topical anesthetics (especially esters such as benzocaine)
    Fragrances
    Lanolin

ERYTHEMA MULTIFORME

<u>Idiopathic</u>

<u>Medications</u> (please see medication reactions)
    Antibiotics (esp. sulfonamides, penicillin, ethosuximide, tetracycline)
    Anti-seizure medications (esp. phenytoin)
    Others

Infectious
    Viral (esp. recurrent HSV, also EBV, Coxsackie, echovirus, & influenza)
    Bacterial (Francisella, Yersinia)
    Chlamydia (LGV)
    Mycoplasma pneumoniae
    Fungal
    Parasitic (malaria, Trichomonas)
Vaccines (BCG, polio, smallpox)
Neoplasms (Lymphoma, carcinoma)
Hematologic disorders (Leukemia, multiple myeloma, polycythemia vera)
Physical agents
    Rhus dermatitis (poison oak, ivy, or sumac)
    Radiation

ERYTHEMA NODOSUM
Idiopathic
Infectious
    Bacterial
        Streptococci, also Yersinia, B. henselae, Salmonella, Campylobacter,
        M. pneumonia, Tularemia
    Fungal
        Histoplasmosis, Coccidioidomycosis, Blastomycosis, Trichophyton
    Mycobacterial
        Tuberculosis, Leprosy
    Leptospirosis
    Chlamydial
        LGV, psittacosis
    Viral
        hepatitis
Medications
    OCPs, please see medication reactions for other
Systemic
    Sarcoidosis
    Behçet's syndrome
    Inflammatory bowel disease
Hematologic
    Leukemia
    Lymphoma
Radiation therapy
Pregnancy

ERYTHRODERMA (mnemonic DI-SCALPP)
Drug (please see medication reactions)
Idiopathic
Seborrheic dermatitis
Contact dermatitis
Atopic dermatitis
Lymphoma (especially CTCL/Sézary syndrome)
Pityriasis rubra pilaris
Psoriasis

HAND DERMATITIS (HAND ECZEMA)
Excessive hand washing
Cold air
Low humidity
Atopic dermatitis
Dyshidrotic eczema
Psoriasiform dermatitis
Contact dermatitis
Allergic dermatitis
Pityriasis rubra pilaris
Keratolysis exfoliativa

HIRSUTISM
<u>Idiopathic</u>
<u>Medications</u>
 Anabolic steroids
 Oral contraceptives (rare with low dose)
 Other
<u>Endocrinopathies</u>
 ACTH excess
 Adrenogenital syndrome
 Adrenal (hyperplasia, adenoma, carcinoma)
 Pituitary tumor (Cushing's disease, acromegaly, prolactinoma)
 Polycystic ovarian disease
 Ovarian hyperthecosis
 Ovarian tumor
 Insulin resistance
 HAIR-AN syndrome

HYPERTRICHOSIS
<u>Hypertrichosis lanuginosa</u>
 Congenital
 Acquired ("malignant down")
<u>Nutrition</u> (anorexia, malnutrition)
<u>Medications</u>
 Minoxidil
 Phenytoin
 Diazoxide
 Cyclosporine
 Oral corticosteroids
 Penicillamine
<u>Syndromes</u>
 Porphyrias (PCT, VP)
 Mucopolysaccharidoses (esp. Hurler's)
 Cornelia de Lange's syndrome
 Morquio's disease
 Leprechaunism

HYPERPIGMENTATION

Primary
   Localized
      Ephelides (freckles)
      Acanthosis nigricans
      Seborrheic keratosis
      Café au lait spots
      Pigmented actinic keratosis
      Lentigo
      Nevus
      Melanoma
      Dermal melanosis (Mongolian spot)

Systemic diseases
   Localized
      Acanthosis nigricans
         Idiopathic
         Endocrine disorders
         Paraneoplastic
      Lentigines
      Peutz-Jeghers syndrome
      LEOPARD syndromes
      Xeroderma pigmentosum
      Carney complex
      Café au lait spots
      Urticaria pigmentosa
      Dyskeratosis congenita
   Diffuse
      Metabolic
      Porphyria cutanea tarda
      Hemochromatosis
      Endocrinopathies
         Addison's disease
         Nelson's syndrome
         Ectopic ACTH syndrome
      Malabsorption
         Whipple's disease (frequent, photodistribution)
      Metastatic melanoma (with melanosis)
      Autoimmune
         Biliary cirrhosis
         Scleroderma
         POEMS syndrome
   Medications   see Medication reactions (pigmentation reactions)

HYPOPIGMENTATION/DEPIGMENTATION

Vitiligo
Chemical leukoderma
Piebaldism
Tinea versicolor
Post inflammatory hypopigmentation
Oculocutaneous albinism   (Hypopigmentation continued)

Hermansky-Pudlak syndrome
Chédiak-Higashi syndrome
Vogt-Koyanagi-Harada
Scleroderma
Halo surrounding pigmented lesion
Tuberous sclerosis (ash leaf spot)
Hypomelanosis of Ito/mosaicism
Nevus anemicus
Nevus depigmentosus
Sarcoidosis
Leprosy
CTCL (Cutaneous T-cell Lymphoma)
Poliosis

MACULOPAPULAR GENERALIZED ERUPTION

<u>Medications</u>
  see medication reactions
  Antibiotics and others
<u>Graft-versus-host disease</u>
<u>Infectious</u>
  Viral
    Rubeola
    Rubella
    Roseola (HHV-6)
    Erythema infectiosum (parvovirus B19)
    EBV
    Cytomegalovirus
    Hepatitis B
    Adenovirus
    Enterovirus
    Reovirus
    Arbovirus
    Rhabdovirus
    HIV
    Live viral vaccine (measles)
  Bacterial
    Streptococcal
    Staphylococcal
    Salmonella
    Meningococcemia
  Mycoplasma
  Secondary syphilis
  Leptospirosis
  Spirillum minus
  Rickettsial
  Psittacosis
  Toxoplasmosis
  Leprosy
  Trichinosis

MEDICATION REACTIONS:

ALOPECIA
ACE inhibitors
Allopurinol
Anticoagulants
Antithyroid drugs
Antineoplastic agents
  (anagen effluvium)
Anti-seizure medications
Beta-blockers
Colchicine
Hypocholesteremic drugs
Indomethacin
Levodopa
OCP
Quinacrine
Retinoids
  (etretinate, isotretinoin, etc.)
Thallium
Vitamin A

ACNEIFORM/PUSTULAR
Bromides/iodides
Androgens
Anabolic steroids
Corticosteroids
Oral contraceptives
Isoniazid
Lithium
Phenobarbital
Phenytoin

ANAPHYLACTIC REACTION
Aspirin
Penicillin
Radiographic dye
Serum (animal)
Tolmetin

Bullous lesions (see vesicles/blisters)

ERYTHEMA MULTIFORME
Sulfa medications
  (sulfonamides, dapsone, etc.)
Allopurinol
Barbiturates
Carbamazepine
Minoxidil
Nitrofurantoin

Nonsteroidal anti-inflammatory agents
Penicillin
Phenolphthalein
Phenothiazines
Phenytoin
Rifampin
Sulfonamides
Sulfonylureas
Sulindac

ERYTHEMA NODOSUM
Bromides/Iodides
Oral contraceptives
Sulfonamides
Penicillin and derivatives

EXFOLIATIVE ERYTHRODERMA
ACE inhibitors
  (captopril)
Allopurinol
Arsenic
Barbiturates
Cefoxitin
Chloroquine
Cimetidine
Gold salts
Isoniazid
Lithium
Mercurial diuretics
Paraaminosalicylic acid
Phenylbutazone
Phenytoin
Sulfonamides
Sulfonylureas

FIXED DRUG REACTIONS
(local, non-spreading,, recur when
  rechallenged with same drug)
Antibiotics: tetracycline, minocycline,
  sulfonamides, metronidazole, nystatin
Anti-inflammatory medications
  NSAIDs, ASA, phenylbutazone,
  AND phenacetin
Sedative/hypnotics
  barbiturates, methaqualone, etc
OCP
Phenolphthalein
Quinine
Many others

MEDICATION REACTIONS (cont'd)

LICHEN PLANUS-LIKE ERUPTIONS

ACE inhibitors (captopril)
Antimalarials
Arsenic
Beta-blockers
Diuretics (furosemide)
Gold salts
Methyldopa
Penicillamine
Quinidine
Sulfonylureas
Thiazides

MACULOPAPULAR/
EXANTHEMATOUS ERUPTIONS

Ampicillin (esp. with mononucleosis)
Barbiturates
Diflunisal (Dolobid)
Gentamicin
Gold salts
Isoniazid
Meclofenamate (Meclomen)
Phenothiazines
Phenylbutazone
Phenytoin
Quinidine
Sulfonamides
Thiazides
Thiouracil
Trimethoprim-sulfamethoxazole
    (in HIV)

PHOTOSENSITIVITY REACTIONS

Amiodarone
Chlorpropamide
Furosemide
Griseofulvin
Lomefloxacin
Methotrexate
Nalidixic acid
Naproxen
Phenothiazines
Piroxicam (Feldene)
Psoralens
Quinine
Sulfonamides
Tetracycline
Thiazides
Tolbutamide

PIGMENTATION REACTIONS

ACTH
    Addisonian pigmentation
Amiodarone
    Slate-gray in photodistribution
Antimalarials
    Blue oral mucosa and pretibial
Argyria
    (Silver containing meds)
    Blue-gray skin from nose drops or
    sulfadiazine
Bleomycin
    Brown to black linear pigmentation
    and post-dermatographism
Busulfan
    Hyperpigmentation (like Addison's)
Carotene
    Yellow/Orange discoloration
Chlorpromazine
    Brown, blue, or slate-gray in a
    photodistribution
Chrysiasis
    (Gold containing meds)
    Red to violet in photodistribution
Clofazimine
    Pink to black excretory products
    and skin in a photodistribution
Cyclophosphamide
    Macular to diffuse brown
Estrogen/progestins
    Melasma
Iron
    Local or generalized brown to gray
    discoloration from iron injections
Minocycline
    Blue to gray stippling on extensor
    surfaces, trauma sites, oral mucosa,
    teeth, face, bones, thyroid
Phenytoin
    Patches of hyperpigmentation
    similar to melasma
Zidovudine
    Brown macules on oral mucosa/lips
    and brown lines in fingernails

MEDICATION REACTIONS (cont'd)

PIGMENTED PURPURIC
ERUPTIONS (capillaritis)
HCTZ
Carbromal
Meprobamate
NSAIDS
Acetaminophen
Ampicillin

PITYRIASIS ROSEA LIKE
ACE inhibitors (captopril)
Arsenic
Barbiturates
Bismuth
Clonidine
Gold salts
Methoxypromazine
Metronidazole
Pyribenzamine

STEVENS JOHNSON SYNDROME
(50% are drug-related)
Carbamazepine
Phenytoin
Phenobarbital
Sulfonamides
Penicillins
Many other

TOXIC EPIDERMAL NECROLYSIS
(80% are drug-related)
Allopurinol
Phenylbutazone
Phenytoin
Sulfonamides
Sulindac

VASCULITIS Cutaneous Small Vessels
Acetaminophen
Allopurinol
Ampicillin
HCTZ
Hydralazine
Meprobamate
Penicillin
Piroxicam
Propylthiouracil
Quinidine
Sulfonamides

VESICLES/BLISTERS
Bromides/Iodides
Cicatricial pemphigoid-like
    Clonidine
PCT-like
    Naproxen
Pemphigus-like
    ACE inhibitor (captopril)
    Cephalosporins
    Penicillamine
Phototoxic/photoallergic
    Furosemide
    Piroxicam
Pressure-related
    Barbiturates
    Sulfonamides

21

MUCOSAL LESIONS
Aphthous ulcers
Behçet's syndrome (recurrent ulcers)
Bullous pemphigoid
Candida
Erythema multiforme
Cicatricial pemphigoid
Hand-foot-and-mouth disease
Herpangina
Herpes gingivostomatitis (primary)
Lichen planus
Medications (fixed drug reaction, chemotherapy, anti-neoplastic agents, gold)
Mucocele
Pemphigus vulgaris
Reiter's syndrome
Sjögren's syndrome
Squamous cell carcinoma
Stevens-Johnson syndrome
Submucosal fibroma

NAIL-PITTING
Alopecia areata
Psoriasis
Koilonychia

PAPULO-NODULAR
Flesh-colored
    Angiofibromas
    Basal cell epitheliomas
    Epidermal cysts and pilar cysts
    Lipomas (soft)
    Molluscum contagiosum
    Neurofibromas
    Neuromas
    Rheumatoid nodule
    Skin tags
    Syringoma
    Tricholemmomas
Pink/translucent colored
    Amyloidosis
    Papular mucinosis
White-colored
    Calcinosis cutis
    Milium
Yellow-colored
    Necrobiosis lipoidica
    Pseudoxanthoma elasticum
    Sebaceous adenomas
    Tophi
    Xanthomas and xanthelasma

PAPULO-NODULAR - (cont'd)

Red/Pink colored
   Papules
      Angiofibromas
      Angiokeratomas
      Arthropod bites
      Bacillary angiomatosis
      Cherry hemangiomas
      Pyogenic granuloma (lobular capillary hemangioma)
   Papules/plaques
      Cutaneous lupus
      Granuloma annulare
      Lymphocytoma cutis (pseudolymphoma)
      Lymphoma cutis
      Leukemia cutis
      Polymorphous light eruption
   Nodules
      Cutaneous metastases
      Keratoacanthoma/Squamous cell carcinoma

Red-brown colored
   Bowenoid papulosis
   Erythema elevatum diutinum (chronic leukocytoclastic vasculitis)
   Lupus vulgaris
   Sarcoidosis
   Urticaria pigmentosa

Blue-colored
   Blue nevus
   Dermatofibroma
   Glomus tumor
   Primary or metastatic melanoma
   Venous lake
   Venous malformations (blue rubber bleb syndrome)

Violaceous
   Cutaneous lupus
   Lichen Planus
   Lupus pernio (sarcoidosis)
   Lymphoma cutis

Purple-colored
   Angiosarcoma
   Kaposi's sarcoma
   Palpable purpura (vasculitis)

Brown-black colored
   see "Hyperpigmentation"

NOTE:
If the papule or nodule is hard/firm, consider Cutaneous Metastases which is often skin colored, pink, red, or brown.

PAPULOSQUAMOUS ERUPTIONS
Actinic keratosis
Lichen planus
Lichen simplex chronicus
Lichen striatus
Pellagra (greasy scaling dermatitis of face, ears, vulva, scrotum, etc.)
Pityriasis lichenoides chronica/PLEVA
Pityriasis rosea
Pityriasis rubra pilaris
Psoriasis
Eczema
Seborrheic dermatitis
Secondary Syphilis
Crusted scabies

PARANEOPLASTIC

SIGN	ASSOCIATED MALIGNANCY
Dermatomyositis	Breast, bronchus
Erythema gyratum repens	Bronchus, ovary, and breast malignancy
Tylosis	Esophageal cancer
Acanthosis nigricans	Gastric cancer
Thrombophlebitis migrans	Pancreatic cancer
Necrolytic migratory erythema	Glucagonoma
Acquired ichthyosis	Lymphoma
Bullous pyoderma gangrenosum	Leukemia/myeloma
Sweet's syndrome	AML/CML
Leser-Trélat	Gastric and adenocarcinomas
Hypertrichosis lanuginosa uterus	Breast, lung, gallbladder, GI, bladder,

PETECHIAL ERUPTIONS
RMSF
Meningococcemia
Echoviruses
Coxsackie
Gonococcemia
Allergic vasculitis

PRURITIC LESIONS

Chronic scratching
  Lichen simplex chronicus
  Prurigo nodularis
Cutaneous
  Atopic dermatitis
  Contact dermatitis
  Eczema
  Seborrheic dermatitis
  Stasis dermatitis
  Urticaria
  Xerosis (dry skin)
    Excess bathing
    Low humidity
  Bullous pemphigoid
  Lichen planus
  Mastocytosis
  Mycosis fungoides
Infectious
  Bacterial
  Fungal
  VZV
Infestations
  Scabies
  Lice
Insect bite reactions
  Fleas, chiggers, ticks, others
HIV
  Eosinophilic folliculitis

PRURITUS WITHOUT LESIONS

Dry skin
  Excessive bathing
  Harsh soaps
  Cold weather
Medications
  Opiates
  Angiotensin-converting enzyme inhibitors
  Sulfonylureas
  Diuretics
  Anticoagulants
  Aspirin
  Quinidine
  Phenothiazine
  Vitamin B
  Estrogen
  Antithyroid medications
  Progesterone
  Androgens
  Others

(Pruritus continued)

Systemic
    Diabetes mellitus
    Hepatobiliary disease (intra & extrahepatic)
        Bile duct obstruction
        Biliary cirrhosis
        Drug-induced cholestasis
        Intrahepatic cholestasis of pregnancy
    HIV
    Chronic renal failure
        Uremia
        Hemodialysis-related
    Hypothyroidism
    Hyperthyroidism
    Medications (chlorpropamide, oral contraceptives, phenothiazine)
Neoplasm
    Lymphoma (esp. Hodgkin's disease)
    Carcinoid
    CNS
    Intestinal
    Gastric
    Pancreatic
    Paraproteinemias (esp. multiple myeloma)
    Polycythemia vera
Neurodermatitis
Dermatographism
Senile pruritus (>70 yo)
Xerosis
Fiberglass exposure

PURPURA/NON-PALPABLE
Medications
        Heparin, Aspirin, Cytotoxic agents, NSAIDS, Ethanol, Estrogen,
        Steroid purpura (topical, <1% oral)
Insecticides
Disseminated intravascular coagulation
    Overwhelming sepsis
    Anaphylaxis
    Neoplasm (lung, prostate, and pancreas cancer, lymphoma, leukemia)
Thrombotic thrombocytopenia purpura
Immune thrombocytopenic purpura
Posttransfusion purpura
Marrow failure
Splenic platelet sequestration
Wiskott-Aldrich syndrome
Platelet dysfunction
    Glanzmann's thrombasthenia
    Von Willebrand's disease
    Thrombocytopenia
Capillaritis
    Pigmented purpuric eruptions

Solar purpura
Trauma
Thrombi
Monoclonal cryoglobulinemia
Warfarin necrosis
Embolic
   Cholesterol
   Fat
   Septic
Systemic
   Amyloidosis
      pinch purpura
   Clotting factor defects
   Ehlers-Danlos syndrome
   Scurvy
   Waldenström's macroglobulinemia
Psychiatric
   Gardner-Diamond syndrome

PURPURA/PALPABLE

Systemic vasculitis
   Polyarteritis nodosa
   Henoch-Schönlein purpura
   Churg-Strauss syndrome
   Wegener's granulomatosis
   Lupus erythematosus
   Rheumatoid arthritis
   Subacute bacterial endocarditis
   Hepatitis B
   Serum sickness
   Cryoglobulinemia
   Sjögren's syndrome
   Hyperglobulinemia
   Waldenström's macroglobulinemia
   Lymphoproliferative disorders (Hodgkin's)
Medications (see medication reactions/vasculitis)
Septic vasculitis
   Acute meningococcemia
   Disseminated gonococcal infection
   RMSF
   Ecthyma gangrenosum

PUSTULAR LESIONS

Acne vulgaris, rosacea
Medications
   see medication reactions/acneiform eruptions
Behçet's syndrome
Polycystic ovary disease
Cushing's disease
Adrenal hyperplasia

RASH WITH FEVER
Drug fever
Pustular psoriasis
Erythroderma
Sweet's syndrome
RMSF

RETICULAR RASH
Cutis marmorata (physiologic)
Erythema ab igne
Livedo reticularis (pathologic)

TELANGIECTASIAS
Acne rosacea
Actinically damaged skin
Venous hypertension
    varicose veins
Polycythemia vera
Essential telangiectasia
Osler-Weber-Rendu syndrome (HHT)
Poikiloderma
    Ionizing radiation
    Poikiloderma vasculare atrophicans (DM, CTCL)
    Xeroderma pigmentosum
Spider angioma
    Idiopathic
    OCP
    Pregnancy
    Cirrhosis
Ataxia-telangiectasia
Mastocytosis (TMEP type)
Scleroderma (CREST)
Periungual
    Lupus
    Scleroderma
    Dermatomyositis
Endocrinopathy
    Estrogen
    Progesterone
    Topical corticosteroids (chronic)
    Hyperthyroidism
    Cirrhosis
Neoplasms
    Breast
    Bile duct
    Carcinoid
    CTCL
    Malignant angioendotheliomatosis

ULCERS
Arterial ulcers
Livedoid vasculitis
Squamous cell carcinoma
Basal cell carcinoma
Pyoderma
Venous ulcers
Pressure
Diabetic
Genital/Sexually transmitted
   Chancroid (exquisite pain)
   Syphilis
   Granuloma inguinale
   LGV
Mucosal
   Behçet's disease
   Erythema multiforme
   Lichen planus
   Pemphigus vulgaris and other autoimmune blistering disorders
   SLE
   Stevens-Johnson syndrome
Systemic
   Antiphospholipid syndrome
   Cholesterol emboli
   Cryofibrinogenemia
   Cryoglobulinemias
   Fungal infection
   Herpes varicella/zoster chronic infection
   Hemoglobinopathies`
   Leukocytoclastic vasculitis
   Lymphoma
   Necrobiosis Lipoidica
   Pyoderma gangrenosum
   Raynaud's disease
   Mycobacterial
   Ecthyma gangrenosum
Medication
   Pentazocine (Talwin)
   IV infiltrate
Factitial

UTRICARIA

<u>Primary</u>
    Idiopathic (most)
    Physical urticaria
        Dermatographism
        Solar urticaria
        Cold urticaria
        Cholinergic urticaria
        Heat urticaria
    Angioedema (hereditary and acquired)
<u>Systemic diseases</u>
    Urticarial vasculitis
    Hepatitis B infection
    Serum sickness
    Angioedema (hereditary and acquired)
    Mastocytosis

VESICULAR/BULLOUS LESIONS

<u>Autoimmune</u>
    Bullous pemphigoid
    Dermatitis herpetiformis
    Epidermolysis bullosa
    Herpes gestationis
    Linear IgA disease
    Pemphigus vulgaris
<u>Infectious</u>
    Bullous impetigo
    Herpes simplex
    Staphylococcal scalded skin syndrome
    Varicella/zoster
<u>Secondary</u>
    Contact dermatitis
    Erythema multiforme
    Toxic epidermal necrolysis
<u>Systemic</u>
    Coma bullae
    Diabetic bullae
    Hemodialysis bullous dermatosis
    Paraneoplastic pemphigus
    Porphyria cutanea tarda
    Pseudoporphyria

5

DERMATOLOGICAL ACRONYMS

AE- Acrodermatitis Enteropathica

ACD- Allergic Contact Dermatitis

BCC- Basal Cell Carcinoma

CAL- Café Au Lait macules

CREST syndrome-
Calcinosis, Raynaud's syndrome, Esophageal dysmotility, Sclerosis, Telangiectasia
Subtype of scleroderma.

CTCL- Cutaneous T-Cell Lymphoma

CTD- Connective Tissue Disorder

DIC- Disseminated Intravascular Coagulation

EM- Erythema Multiforme

EPP- Erythropoietic ProtoPorphyria

GA- Granuloma Annulare

HAIR-AN syndrome-
HyperAndrogenism, Insulin Resistance, and Acanthosis Nigricans

HG- Herpes Gestationis

HHT- Hereditary Hemorrhagic Telangiectasia

HPV- Human Papilloma Virus.

HSV- Herpes Simplex Virus.

ICD- Irritant Contact Dermatitis

LAMB- Lentigines, Atrial Myxoma, Blue nevi.

LEOPARD-
Lentigines, EKG abnormalities, Ocular hypertelorism, Pulmonary stenosis, Abnormal genitalia, Retardation of growth, Deafness.

LP- Lichen Planus

LSA- Lichen Sclerosis et Atrophicus

MF- Mycosis Fungoides

NAME – Nevus, Atrial myxoma, Myxoid neurofibroma, Ephelides.

NF- NeuroFibromatosis

NL- Necrobiosis Lipoidica

PAN- PolyArteritis Nodosa

PCT- Porphyria Cutanea Tarda

PLEVA- pityriasis lichenoides et varioliformis acutis

PMLE- PolyMorphous Light Eruption

POEMS-
Polyneuropathy, Organomegaly, Endocrinopathy, M protein, Skin changes.

PPE- Pigmented Purpuric Eruptions/capillaritis

PUPPP- Pruritic Urticarial Plaques and Papules of Pregnancy

PUVA- Psoralens and UltraViolet A

PV- Pemphigus Vulgaris

PXE- PseudoXanthoma Elasticum

RAST- RadioAllergoSorbent Test

RMSF- Rocky Mountain Spotted Fever

SJS- Steven-Johnson Syndrome

SLE- Systemic Lupus Erythematosus

SSSS or SSS- (Staphylococcal) Scalded-Skin Syndrome.

TEN- Toxic Epidermal Necrolysis

TSS- Toxic Shock Syndrome

TTP- Thrombocytopenia Purpura

VP- Variegate Porphyria

6

USEFUL DERMATOLOGICAL TERMINOLOGY

Acantholysis- separation of keratinocytes due to loss of epidermal cohesion;
   disruption of intercellular bridges of the epidermal spinosum layer.

Acanthosis nigricans- thickened velvety region of hyperpigmentation usually in
   skin folds and axilla; may be benign from obesity, but can also indicate an
   endocrine abnormality or paraneoplastic syndrome.

Acne rosacea- chronic skin eruptions characterized by flushing and eventually
   telangiectasias and rhynophyma.

Acne vulgaris (common acne)- pilosebaceous inflammation from hormonal and
   bacterial influences (Propionobacterium acnes).

Acral lentiginous melanoma-cutaneous melanoma located on palm, fingernail,
   sole, toenail, and mucous membranes, more common in Asians and Africans.

Acrochordon- skin tag.

Acrodermatitis- dermatitis of the face, hands, feet, and anogenital region.

Acrodermatitis enteropathica- zinc deficiency, malabsorption or dietary, characterized by dry pink erosive patches usually involving hands, feet, and anogenital
   regions and associated with diarrhea and alopecia.

Acrosclerosis- sclerosis of the hands that may be associated with necrosis and
   ulceration of the fingertips.

Actinic keratosis (solar keratosis)-scaling macules on sun-exposed skin, often tender.

Albright's syndrome- precocious puberty, polyostotic fibrous dysplasias,
   café au lait macules.

Alopecia- hair loss.

Alopecia areata- localized hair loss often associated with an autoimmune disease.

Amyloidosis - abnormal deposition of amyloid protein in various tissues.

Anergy skin test - inappropriate decreased immune reactivity to skin tests, e.g.,
   PPD in immunocompromised patient with prior positive test.

Angiofibromata- small erythematous papules that arise on the lower face of
   children with tuberous sclerosis.

Angiokeratoma- term used to describe many distinct conditions of vascular and
   keratotic lesions.

Angioedema- transient vascular reaction within deep dermis that results in pruritic
   localized dermal edema due to dilation and increased permeability of capillaries
   similar to urticaria.

Angiosarcoma- malignant vascular neoplasm.

Annular - ring shaped.

Aphthous ulcers (canker sores)- painful oral ulcerations of unknown etiology, usually occur in the mouth but may also involve the anus, genitalia, or gastrointestinal tract.

Arciform - bow shaped.

Ash-leaf spots- oval white macules in patients with tuberous sclerosis.

Asteatotic eczema- xerotic eczema or "winter itch." Dry, fissured, erythematous lesions over the shins, hands, arms and trunks of elderly persons, which is usually secondary to excessive bathing.

Athlete's foot- see tinea pedis.

Atopic dermatitis/eczema (eczema, IgE dermatitis)- pruritic dry skin condition commonly occurring in arm and leg flexures, dorsa of wrists and feet, face, neck, and eyelids often heritable condition of pruritus followed by rash associated with history of asthma or seasonal allergies. "The itch that rashes."

Atrophie blanche- shiny, white, stippled scars on ankle or foot due to chronic venous insufficiency.

Atrophic- wasting away of tissue or organ.

Auspitz's sign- plaques of psoriasis reveal bleeding points when scale removed. Not specific for psoriasis.

Bacilliary angiomatosis- widely distributed red papules occurring in patients with HIV who have been scratched by a cat (*Bartonella*).

Basal cell carcinoma- most common cancer. It is locally invasive, characterized by pearly papules or nodules.

Basal cell epithelioma- see Basal cell carcinoma.

Bazin's disease- nodular vasculitis associated with *Mycobacterium tuberculosis*.

Beau's lines- transverse line across nail plate, signifies arrested nail growth due to stress or illness.

Becker's nevus- pigmented hamartoma which occurs more commonly on shoulder of males in their teens. It commonly grows hair within 1 year.

Behçet's syndrome- multisystem disorders characterized by recurrent oral aphthous ulcers and 2 of the following: recurrent genital aphthous ulcers, posterior uveitis, erythema nodosum, or cutaneous pustular vasculitis.

Blancheable - pallor or loss of color upon compression.

Blister - vesicle or bulla occurring between epidermis and dermis or within dermis.

Blood Blister - blister filled with blood usually result of pinching trauma to skin.

Boil- skin abscess.

Bowen's disease- squamous cell carcinoma in-situ.

Bowenoid papulosis- slow growing pigmented macule in anogenital region, histologically similar to squamous cell carcinoma in situ but often occurring at multiple sites.

Bruise - see ecchymosis.

Bullae - fluid filled cystic structure > 0.5 cm.

Bullous pemphigoid- autoimmune tense mucocutaneous bullae characterized by neutrophils in dermal-epidermal junction with IgG along basement membrane.

Burn 1st Degree - involves superficial epidermis.

Burn 2nd Degree - involves epidermis and papillary dermis associated with blister formation and pain.

Burn 3rd Degree - destruction of all derma layers, typically not associated with pain due to destruction of nerve endings.

Burrow -sinus or fistula furrowed into the skin by a parasite.

33

Café aulait macules- large tan to brown macules which may be found in high
    numbers in patients affected with Albrights's syndrome or Neurofibromatosis.
    Benign lesions of melanin macroglobules.

Calciphylaxis - small/medium vessel calcification with progressive cutaneous
    necrosis, associated with end-stage renal disease and hyperparathyroidism.

Callus- local region of hyperkeratosis caused by chronic use and pressure.

Canities - graying or whitening of hair from normal aging.

Canities unguium - white spots or white streaks beneath the nails.

Canker sores- see aphthous ulcer.

Carbuncle- inflammatory nodules or abscess of numerous contiguous hair follicles.

Cellulitis - diffuse inflammation of subcutaneous connective tissue.

Cerebreform - morphology resembling the surface of the brain.

Chalazion (stye) - any inflammatory process involving the eyelash hair follicle.

Chancroid- painful ulceration usually appearing on external genitalia following
    sexual transmission of *Hemophilus ducreyi*.

Chapped lips - dry, fissured epidermis of lips commonly related to dehydration or
    low environmental temperatures.

Chédiak-Higashi syndrome- albinism associated with thrombocytopenia and
    repeated bacterial infections.

Cheilitis- inflammation of the lips.

Cheilosis - fissuring of the lips and angles of the mouth especially with
    riboflavin deficiency.

Cherry angioma- papules or nodules composed of small blood vessels.

Chicken pox - papulovesicular eruptions during acute VZV infection.

Chloasma- melasma.

Chloroma- yellow-green ulcerated tumor associated with leukemia cutis.

Chronoaging - normal aging process of skin that results in wrinkling, decreased
    skin thickness, decreased metabolic activity, decreased collagen synthesis,
    degeneration of elastin fibers, and decrease in glycosominoglycans.

Cicatrix - scar.

Clarks nevus- dysplastic melanocytic nevus.

Cold sores - recurrent vesicular lesions of HSV infection of lips.

Comedones- blackheads or whiteheads; keratin/sebum plug in a hair follicle.

Condyloma lata- pink-brown flat-topped papules; appear with secondary syphilis.

Condyloma accuminata- genital verruca (wart) caused by HPV.

Conjunctivitis - inflammation of conjunctiva, usually contagious from infection,
    but could be allergic reaction or other.

Contact dermatitis (eczematous dermatitis)- allergic (type IV) reaction to agents
    such as poison ivy (Rhus dermatitis), mango peel, metals, etc.

Corium- dermis.

Cowden's disease- also known as multiple hamartoma syndrome is an autosomal
    dominant syndrome characterized by multiple skin findings and an association
    with internal malignancy.

Crab lice- pubic hair infestation with *Phthirus pubis* lice.

Crust - dried liquid debris (puss or serous fluid) that has been deposited on the
    surface of skin.

Cutis - skin.

Cutis anserina - "Goose Flesh," "Goose Pimples," the skins appearance upon
    contraction of arrectores pilorum muscles (in response to cold or emotions).

Cutis marmorata- vascular anomaly characterized by a bluish or purple reticular appearance and often associated with other congenital abnormalities.

Cyst - vesicle filled with liquid or semi-solid material, located between dermis and epidermis.

Dandruff - dry, scaly desquamation of scalp epidermis.

Decubitus ulcer - ulceration that occurs at pressure points due to immobilization and chronic pressure maybe superficial or very deep.

Darier's sign- characteristic of cutaneous mastocytosis, a wheal develops at site of pressure applied from a blunt instrument. Secondary to mast cell degranulation.

Darling's disease- histoplasmosis.

Dennie-morgan folds/lines- infraorbital folds associated with hyperpigmentation and hyperkeratosis in atopic individuals.

Dercum's disease- multiple painful lipomas arising in adulthood.

Dermatitis herpetiformis- recurrent pruritic cluster of vesicles on an erythematous base located on extensor surfaces.

Dermatographism- urticarial lesion at site of firmly stroked skin, more common in patients with chronic urticaria.

Dermatofibroma- firm red, blue, brown nodule that dimples with lateral pressure.

Dermatoheliosis- photo aging.

Dermatomyositis- heliotrope rash encircling eyes, associated with an erythematous rash on face, neck, and shoulders in a "shawl-like" distribution.

Dermatophytosis- annular, scaly patch of infection with Epidermophyton, Trichophyton, or Microsporum.

Dermoid cyst - present at birth in skin along lines of embryonic fusion, caused by disruption during embryogenesis; contains skin elements including hair.

Desmoplasia- connective tissue proliferation.

Desquamation - casting off of epidermis and scales or sheets.

Diascopy- firm pressure of microscope slide over skin lesion.

Discoid lupus- telangiectatic, dyspigmented, lesions with follicular plugging that are rarely (<5%) associated with systemic disease.

Dyshidrotic eczema- deep-seated, pruritic, burning, clear blisters located on palms and soles. "Tapioca pudding." Caused by atopy or contact dermatitis.

Dysplastic nevus syndrome (Clarks nevus)- acquired nevi; atypical melanocytes; considered by some to be melanoma precursors.

Ecchymosis (bruise) - blue black appearance on skin due to effusion of blood into hypodermis areolar tissue.

Eczema- see atopic dermatitis.

Ecthyma- superficial bacterial infection with extension into the dermis, more common on lower extremities and characterized by ulcerations.

Edema (pitting) - excessive fluid in the interstitial space.

Edema (non-pitting) - see myxevema.

Elastosis - disorder of elastic fibers.

Ephelides- freckles, see pigmented lesions.

Epidermal inclusion cyst- type of epidermoid cyst, which is caused by traumatic introduction of epidermal components into the dermis.

Epidermoid cyst (sebaceous cyst, epidermal cyst, wen, infundibular cyst)- epithelium components such as keratin and lipid-laden debris produced by a hair follicle which becomes entrapped in the dermis.

Epidermolysis bullosa- a collection of autosomal dominant and recessive bullous diseases characterized immunologically by type IV collagen, laminin, or pemphigoid antibodies in the bullae.

Erosion- lesion characterized by loss of the epidermis only, see ulcer.

Eruption - breakout of a rash on the skin.

Erysipelas- painful, edematous, well-demarcated erythematous eruption caused by streptococcal infection, usually with fever and other constitutional symptoms.

Erythematous - redness of the skin due to hyperemia.

Erythema ab igne- reticulated, hyperpigmented regions associated with chronic heat exposure (heating pads, radiator, fireplace).

Erythema annulare centrificum- impetigo presenting in an annular configuration, unlike tinea corporis, vesicles and crusts appear within the ring.

Erythema elevatum diutinum- cutaneous leukocytoclastic vasculitis characterized by a symmetrical distribution of yellow to red papules, plaques, or nodules over the extremities.

Erythema gyratum repens- diabetes related or paraneoplastic phenomenum characterized by granuloma annulare appearing diffusely over the body.

Erythema marginatum- lesions with an erythematous border that are associated with rheumatic fever.

Erythema migrans- (erythema chronicum migrans)- erythematous plaque occurring at the site of the Lyme tick (*Ixodes scapularis)* bite. An annular macule occurs subsequently, due to infection with *Borrelia burgdorferi*. Pathognomonic for Lyme disease.

Erythema multiforme syndrome- erythematous macular or papular target lesions that initially arise in the distal extremeties and migrate centrally, associated with systemic reaction.

Erythema nodosum- painful, erythematous nodules on lower legs due to immunologic/inflammatory response.

Erythroderma- diffuse erythema and hyperkeratosis associated with fever, lymphadenopathy, and generalized systemic reaction.

Erythroplasia of Queyrat- Bowen's disease located on genitalia.

Erythrasma- chronic *Corynebacterium minutissimum* infection that resembles dermatophytosis, and fluoresces coral red on Wood's light exam.

Erythropoietic protoporphyria- porphyria that manifests as a burning sensation on sun exposure and is not associated with an increased excretion of porphyrins.

Eschar - dry scab.

Exantham - skin eruption caused by action of infectious microorganisms or their toxins on skin blood vessels.

Excoriation - breaking away of superficial layers of skin due to scratching or scrapping.

Exfoliation - skin peeling off in scales or sheets.

Exfoliative erythroderma- generalized erythema and desquamation associated with generalized lymphadenopathy and fever due to systemic toxicity. In fixed drug reaction, there are solitary or multiple localized eruptions following ingestion of drug; these recur in the same location upon rechallenge with the same drug.

Fibroma- skin-colored nodule characterized by fibrous or fully differentiated connective tissue.

Fissure - a linear tear in epidermis.

Freckles- ephelides- see pigmented lesions.

Folliculitis- bacterial infection of the hair follicles often caused by *S. aureus*.

Furuncle- tender, nodular infection involving one hair follicle.

Ganglionic cyst - bone cyst lined with membrane filled with fluid, common at dorsum of hand and wrist.

Geographic tongue- benign disorder characterized by hyperkeratosis of the tongue, which may be associated with psoriasis.

Glomus body- arteriole-venule shunt units located in fingertips, face, and ears.

Glomus tumor- glomus body tumor characterized by an intermittently painful subungual papule or nodule.

Glucagonoma syndrome- necrolytic migratory erythema, this annular eruption with peripheral blistering erosions and desquamation is associated with a glucagon secreting pancreatic tumor.

Gluteal pinking- smooth erythematous region in the gluteal fold, associated with seborrheic dermatitis and psoriasis.

Goose-pimples - see Cutis anserina.

Gottron's papules- violaceous/erythematous nodules/plaques at bony prominences associated with dermatomyositis. Observed mostly over MP, PIP, DIP joints.

Gougerot-Blum disease- pigmented purpuric lichenoid dermatitis.

Granuloma - tumor composed of granulation tissue.

Granuloma annulare- asymptomatic papules in an annular arrangement.

Granuloma inguinale - granulomatous ulceration of skin in the genital or inguinal area associated with *Donovania granulomatosis*.

Grover's disease- pruritic transient, papular to vesicular crops of acantholytic dermatosis most commonly occurring in middle-aged men.

Guttate psoriasis- abrupt eruption of psoriatic papules often associated with Streptococcal pharyngitis.

Hand-foot-and- mouth-disease- vesicular eruption of mucous membranes, palms, and soles often associated with viral-like illness caused by Coxsackie virus A16 and occasionally other Coxsackie or Enterviruses.

Hand-Schüller-Christian disease- Langerhans cell histiocytosis.

Hansen's disease- leprosy.

Heberden's nodes - hard nodules at the distal interphalangeal joint of fingers; calcific spurs of articular cartilage in osteoarthritis.

Hemorrhoids- varicose veins of the rectum, which occasionally thrombose and may be painful if external.

Herald patch - the initial lesion in pityriasis rosea; precedes the general eruption.

Hereditary hemorrhagic telangiectasia- autosomal dominant telangiectasias of the skin, mouth, and GI tract.

Hermansky-Pudlak syndrome- albinism associated with defective platelets and bleeding diathesis.

Herpes labialis- sexually transmitted vesicular eruption of the mouth previously with HSV-1, however, HSV-2 is becoming equally as common.

Herpes genitalis- sexually transmitted vesicular eruption of genitalia associated with HSV-2 and sometimes HSV-1.

Herpes gestationis- autoimmune polymorphous pruritic blistering eruption of pregnancy and postpartum.

Herpes zoster- unilateral cutaneous vesicular reaction, which is a recurrence of varicella zoster in a dermatomal distribution.

Hirsuitism - abnormal hairiness, especially on women.

Hive (wheal)- usually describes acute urticaria, see urticaria, see wheal.

Hutchinson's sign- proximal nail fold hyperpigmentation in a Caucasian which is suggestive of malignant melanoma.

Hyperkeratosis - hypertrophy of the corneum layer of skin.

Hyperlinear palms - excessive number of skin lines on palm.

Hypermelanosis - excessive deposits of melanin from melanocytes.

Hyperplasia - over growth of tissue due to increase in number of constituent cells.

Hypertrichosis- excessive hair growth.

Hypertrichosis lanuginosa- lack of replacement of white, fine fetal hair with terminal hair.

Hypertrophic - over growth of tissue due to increased size of constituent cells.

Hypomelanism - insufficient supply of melanin to protect skin against UV light of sun; not albinism.

Hypomelanosis - decrease in supply of melanin to skin by melanocytes.

Ichthyosis- a group of hereditary and acquired disorders characterized by patches of hyperkeratotic lesions distributed in a fish-scale pattern.

Id reaction- inflammatory reaction at a site distant from the original lesion.

IgE dermatitis- see atopic dermatitis.

Impetigo- superficial epidermal infection characterized by golden crusting and caused by *Staphylococcus aureus* or group A ß-hemolytic Streptococci.

Induration - the hardening and thickening of tissue.

Infundibular cyst- see epidermoid cyst.

Inverse psoriasis- psoriasis affecting the intertriginous regions.

Integument - skin.

Janeway lesions- nonpainful hemorrhagic or erythematous nodules of macules on the palms and soles of some patients with infective endocarditis.

Jock itch- see tinea cruris.

Kaposi's sarcoma- vascular neoplasia characterized by multiple violaceous edematous lesions involving any organ, associated with HIV disease.

Kawasaki disease- febrile childhood illness characterized by mucocutaneous erythema with desquamation, cervical lymphadenitis, conjunctivitis, coronary artery aneurysms.

Keloid- progressively enlarging, hypertrophic scar; due to overproduction of collagen in dermis during skin repair; more commonly seen in Africans.

Keratoacanthoma- nodule with central crater, resembles squamous cell carcinoma.

Keratolysis exfoliativa- idiopathic condition characterized by palmar and plantar desquamation.

Keratosis pilaris- erythema surrounding papules of keratin-plugged follicles.

Kerion- dermatophyte infection of the scalp that has become boggy and inflamed as a result of a strong immune response to the fungus.

Koebner's phenomenon- skin changes at site of local injury seen in psoriasis.

Koilonychia- also known as spoon nails, hereditary or acquired softened concave nails often associated with chronic iron deficiency anemia.

Koplik spots - red spots with a white speck in the center, located on bucal and linqual mucosa; prodrome to measles.

Kyrle's disease- grouped pruritic keratotic papules/nodules on extremities, trunk, may be inherited or associated with diabetes mellitus or renal insufficiency.

Langerhans cell histiocytosis- group of disorders characterized by cutaneous and bones lesions, multinucleated giant cells, and granulomas with eosinophils.

Lanugo (down) - fine hair on the body of a fetus.

Leiner's disease- seborrheic dermatitis, diarrhea, C5a deficiency, failure to thrive.

Lentigines- brown pigmented macule due to an increased number of melanocytes and increased production of melanin. They do not darken with sun exposure.

Lentigo maligna- variant of melanoma in-situ. Macule occurring at areas of sun exposure in the elderly. Characterized by color variegation, irregular borders.

Leprosy - infection with bacteria mycobacterium leprae; involves skin and superficial nerves, two types: tuberculoid and lepromatous.

Leser-Trélat sign- abrupt onset of generalized, usually inflammatory, seborrheic keratoses that may be associated with gastric and adenocarcinomas.

Letterer-Siwe syndrome- Langerhans cell histiocytosis.

Leukemia cutis- localized or disseminated eruption of pink, tan, brown, or violaceous papules or nodules associated with leukemia manifestation of leukemic cells in the skin.

Leukoderma- depigmentation due to decreased melanin in melanocytes or loss of melanocytes.

Leukoplakia- white plaque, common on oral mucosa, benign but may be precursor to carcinoma.

Lichenified - characterized by a thickened epidermis.

Lichen planus- shiny, violaceus, pruritic, and flat-topped papules and plaques on mucocutaneous surfaces.

Lichen sclerosis et atrophicus- well-delineated sclerotic plaques and papules.

Lichen simplex chronicus- consequence of pruritic disorders due to chronic scratching or rubbing and characterized by plaques of thickened epidermis.

Lichen striatus- a linear lichenoid eruption, usually self-limited, occurs in children.

Lipodermatosclerosis- thickened, tender, and edematous lower legs due to chronic venous insufficiency.

Lipoma- encapsulated benign proliferation of normal adipose cells.

Lisch nodules- pigmented hamartomas of the iris seen only by slit-lamp, associated with NF1.

Livedo reticularis- blue to purple reticular fish-net like pattern of skin mottling. This macular finding is from statis of blood in the superficial venous system. Benign. Similar to cutis marmorata.

Liver spots- see senile lentigo, solar lentigo.

Lupus erythematosus (SLE)- multi-system connective tisue disease associated with "butterfly" malar facial rash.

Lupus pernio- violaceous plaques on the cheeks, earlobes, and nose in patients with sarcoidosis.

Lupus valgaris- erythematous scaling plaque resulting from endogenous spread of tuberculosis, yellow/brown apple-jelly on diascopy.

Lyell's syndrome- toxic epidermal necrolysis.

Lymphocytoma cutis- asymptomatic plaques or nodules located on the head, extremities, earlobe, areola, or scrotum in patients affected with Lyme disease.

Lymphoma cutis- curtaneous lymphoma often characterized by a firm skin-colored or red nodule.

Macule - discoloration of epidermis; not elevated.

Majocchi's disease- purpura annularis telangiectodes, a variant of PPE.

Majocchi's granuloma- dermatophytic infiltration of hair follicles.

Mee's lines- white transverse bands classically associate with arsenic poisoning.

Melanoma- Malignant tumor that arises from the melanocytic system of the skin or other organs which contain melanocytes.

Melasma- hyperpigmented macules in sun-exposed areas, can be associated with hormonal modulation such as in pregnancy or oral contraceptives.

Migratory necrolytic erythema- annular erythematous necrotic and desquamating plaques, which enlarge with a central clearing and are associated with glucogonoma syndrome.

Miliaria - clogging of sweat pores, resulting in pruritic papular erythematous eruptions.

Milium- small epidermal cyst containing keratin.

Mole - any pigmented fleshy or papula growth of skin.

Molluscum contagiosum- papular lesion often with a central umbilication caused by local Poxvirus infection.

Morbilliform - resembling the rash of measles.

Morphea- local cutaneous sclerosis.

Mottled - skin characterized by colored spots or blotches.

Muehrcke's nails- two white narrow transverse bands on the nailbed associated with hypoalbuminosis. They do not grow out with the nail.

Mycosis fungoides- CTCL.

Myxedema (non-pitting edema)- generalized accumulation of hydrophilic mucopolysaccharides in the dermis due to hypothyroidism. Pretibial myxedema is associated with hyperthyroidism.

Necrobiosis lipoidica- well circumscribed, yellow to brown plaques on anterior and lateral legs, often associated with diabetes mellitus.

Neurofibroma- tumor of nerve connective tissue that may include the medullated layer of the nerve fiber.

Neurofibromatosis I, II - inherited disorder characterized by café aulait spots on skin and neurofibromas of the peripheral nervous system (type I) or central nervous system/cranial nerves (type II).

Neuroma- firm, often painful, cutaneous nodule characterized by hypertrophic nervous tissue arranged in disorganized fascicles.

Nevus sebaceus- yellow to orange-colored congenital alopecic plaque that typically occurs on the scalp.

Nevus spilus- see pigmented lesions.

Nikolsky's sign- skin separation induced by minor pressure.

Nodule - large abnormal aggregation of cells in the epidermis (> 0.5 cm in breadth and depth).

Nummular eczema- "coinlike" lesions of eczema. Common on extensor surfaces of the arms and legs.

Ochronosis- rare pigmentation of bones, ligaments, skin, and urine due to abnormal alkaptonuria metabolism.

Onycholysis- separation of nail plate from nail bed.

Onychomycosis- fungal, yeast or mold infection of fingernails or toenails with characteristic hyperkeratosis of nailbeds.

Osler's nodes- painful violaceous subcutaneous nodules on fingers, toes, thenar, and hypothenar eminences seen in 5% of patients with infective endocarditis.

Osler-Weber-Rendu- see hereditary hemorrhagic telangiectasia.

Paget's disease- eczematous patch on breast areola due to local extension of breast cancer or underlying adenocarcinoma in the case of extramammary disease of the axillary and anogenital skin.

Pancreatic panniculitis- erythematous painful nodules associated with pancreatic cancer or inflammation.

Papilliform - resembling multiple papilla or multiple small nipple-like projections.

Papule - small abnormal aggregation of cells in the epidermis (< 0.5 cm in breadth and depth).

Paronychia- painful erythematous eruption surrounding nailbed. Often associated with bacterial or candidal infection.

Patch - macule with some skin surface scaling or wrinkling.

Pathergy- neutrophilic reaction precipitated by trauma in Behçet's syndrome.

Pediculosis capitis- head lice infection.

Pellagra- red to brown discoloration in sun-exposed regions, diarrhea, and psychosis secondary to niacin deficiency.

Perlèche- fissures at the corners of the mouth.

Pemphigus foliaceus - chronic pemphigus characterized by flacid bullae and exfoliation.

Pemphigus vulgaris- autoimmune mucocutaneous flaccid bullous disease characterized by intraepidermal deposition of IgG.

Petichiae - multiple small reddish/purplish pinpoint spots aggregated on skin caused by extravasation of blood under the epidermis.

Peutz-Jeghers syndrome- familial polyposis syndrome characterized by multiple, small lentigines on the lips and oral mucosa that are usually associated with multiple small bowel hamartomas.

Photoaging - accelerated aging of skin due to chronic exposure to UV radiation of sunlight; increased skin thickness with furrowing and wrinkling, increase of elastin fibers, increase in glycosaminoglycans.

Piebaldism - partial albinism.

Pilar cyst- see trichilemmal cyst.

Pimple- see acne vulgaris.

Pitted keratolysis- pitted, hyperkeratinized skin of the plantar foot associated with hyperhidrosis and *Micrococcus sedentaries* infection.

Pityriasis lichenoides chronica- chronic lesions; appear similar to pityriasis rosea.

Pityriasis rosea- erythematous patches with a collarette of scale in a symmetrical distribution especially on the trunk.

Pityriasis rubra pilaris - rare chronic inflammatory disease of skin; pink scaley patches, follicular papules, with features of seborrheic dermatitis and psoriasis.

Pityriasis versicolor- see Tinea versicolor.

Plaque - elevated lesion of superficial epidermis >0.5 cm breadth, but without significant depth.

Plummer-Vinson syndrome- associated with anemia in middle-aged women and characterized by dysphagia, glossitis, and koilonychia.

Poison ivy-see contact dermatitis.

Poison oak- see contact dermatitis.

Poison sumac- see contact dermatitis.

Poikiloderma- mottled appearance of skin secondary to pigmentary and atrophic change.

Poikiloderma vasculare atrophicans- Can be hypo- or hyperpigmented, wrinkled, and telangiectatic.

Poliosis - irregular patch of white hair on head; benign.

Polyarteritis nodosa- multisystem necrotizing vasculitis of small/medium arteries.

Polymorphis light eruption- group of photodermatoses characterized by erythematous papules and vesicles in response to ultraviolet radiation.

Pompholyx- dyshidrotic eczema.

Porphyria cutanea tarda- bullae/vesicles especially on dorsa of hands; associated with porphyria.

Prickly heat - see Miliaria.

Prurigo nodularis- neurodermatitis characterized by firm pruritic nodules.

Pruritus- itchiness.

Pseudoporphyria- therapy-induced (hemodialysis, drugs, etc) condition mimicking PCT characterized by bullae on dorsa of hands. Porphyrin levels are normal.

Psoriasis- white to silver scaling plaques mostly on extensor surfaces.

Pseudoxanthoma elasticum- hereditary elastic tissue disorder characterized by groups of yellow papules on neck, axillae, and skin folds, GI hemorrhage, hypertension, and angioid streaks in the retina.

Punctate - highly circumscribed like a point.

Purpura - small purplish spots on skin caused by hemorrhage at junction between dermis and hypodermis; larger than petichiae, smaller than eccymosis.

Purpura fulminans - non-thrombocytopenic purpura in children following an infectious disease; can progress to gangrene.

Pustule - vesicle filled with puss.

Pyoderma gangrenosum- rapidly growing ulcer; necrotic base; violaceous overhanging borders; usually associated with ulcerative colitis.

Pyogenic granuloma- fast growing hemangioma, usually caused by minor trauma.

Reiter's syndrome- non-gonococcal urethritis or cervicitis, greater than one month of peripheral arthritis, and frequently keratoderma blennorrhagicum, conjunctivitis, stomatitis, circinate balanitis.

Rosacea- telangiectasias, erythema, papules and pustules on the face.

Rhinophyma- thick erythematous bulbous nose; seen rarely in acne rosacea.

Rhus dermatitis- from contact with plants in the genus *Rhus*: poison ivy, poison oak, poison sumac; they contain a highly allergenic oleoresin called urushiol.

Rhytides - wrinkles.

Ring worm - fungal infection of skin; tends to occur in a circular or ring-like pattern of patches or scale; see tinea corporis.

Sarcoidosis- chronic multisystem granulomatous diseases affecting primarily the skin, lungs, and eyes. Skin lesions are firm, brown–red plaques.

Satellite papules- erythematous papules located at periphery of cutaneous candida infection.

Scab - crust at the site of wound healing.

Scabes- pruritic infestation by mite called *Sarcoptes scabiei*.

Scalded skin syndrome- *S. aureus* exotoxin-induced spreading erythema, which is eventually characterized by painful desquamation, more common in infants.

Scale - thickened stratum corneum that becomes white and dry and flakes off.

Scar - fibrous connective tissue replacement of mesodermal and ectodermal tissue that has been destroyed by injury or disease.

Schamberg's disease- progressive pigmented purpuric eruption typically on legs.

Scleroderma- multisystem progressive sclerosis.

Sclerotic - extensive hardening induration of interstitial substance of a tissue.

Scurvey - vitamin C deficiency resulting in mucocutaneous hemorrhages, spongy gums, and other findings from disruption of collagen synthesis.

Sebaceous adenoma- benign epithelial tumor containing sebum.

Sebaceous cyst- see epidermoid cyst.

Sebaceous hyperplasia- common, small, pink/yellow benign lesions with central umbilication occurring primarily on the face.

Seborrheic dermatitis- chronic erythema/scaling in regions with high concentration of sebaceous glands.

Seborrheic keratosis- verrucous or velvety benign macules or plaques that develop in older individuals. May be benign or sign of systemic malignancy.

Senile lentigo (liver spots)- see solar lentigo.

Sézary syndrome- CTCL characterized by elevated WBC > 20,000/ul (leukemic form with mostly Sézary cells), lymphadenopathy, erythroderma, pruritus, and hair loss.

Shagreen patches- flesh-colored plaques on back and buttocks in patients with Tuberous sclerosis.

Shingles- dermatomal recurrence of *Varicella zoster* virus infection, characterized by burning pain which often preceeds a vesicular erruption.

Simian crease - palm with only one single line, characteristic of Down Syndrome.

Sneddon's syndrome- livedo reticularis associated with hypertension, transient ischemic attacks, and cerebrovascular accidents.

Solar keratosis- erythematous papules and macules with adherent scale due to excess sun exposure.

Solar lentigo- benign macules on areas of chronic sun-exposed skin in elderly, fair skinned individuals. Freckle-like melanosis, but these do not darken with exposure to light. Most common on back of hand, and on forehead.

Splinter hemorrhages- brownish-red streaks in the nail bed that may be caused by trauma or endocarditis.

Spitz nevus- rapidly growing pink or tan nodule, commonly occurs in children.

Stasis ulcer - lower extremity ulcer due to venous stasis or venous insufficiency.

Steatoma - sebaceous cyst.

Steatocystoma - keratin cyst.

Steatocystoma multiplex - rare hereditary disease of multiple sebaceous cyst occurring on trunk and limbs.

Stellate - shaped like a star.

Stevens-Johnson syndrome- mucocutaneous erosions, erythema, and usually <10% exfoliation as a result of a medication or illness. Most common in children and young adults and is associated with a prodrome of high fever, sore throat, cough and other URI symptoms.

Stomatitis- mouth inflammation.

Stye - see Chalazion.

Sunburn - dermatitis associated with redness and blistering of skin caused by exposure to UV rays of sunlight.

Sweet's syndrome- acute febrile neutrophilic dermatosis characterized by painful, erythematous, edematous plaques (esp. neck and upper chest).

Syringoma- intradermal benign eccrine duct adenoma.

Target - ring shaped or multiple concentric ring shaped lesions.

Tarsal cyst - see Chalazion.

Telangiectasia (spider angioma, vascular spider)- red hairline vessels emanating from superficial arteriole-containing papule, may be related to estrogen excess.

Terry's nails- also known as "half and half" nails; the proximal two-thirds of the nailbed is white. They are classically associated with hepatic cirrhosis.

Thrombocytopenic purpura- petechiae and ecchymoses appearing as manifestation of immune and non-immune-mediated thrombocytopenia.

Thrombophlebitis migrans- thrombophlebitis involving different vessels usually simultaneously.

Tinea capitis- hyperkeratotic region of alopecia and broken hairs associated most commonly with *T. tonsurans*, but also with *M. canis*, *M audouinii*, *M. gypseum*, *T. mentagrophytes*, or *T. rubrum*.

Tinea corporis (ringworm)- dematophyte infection involving the trunk, arms, or legs caused by *T. rubrum, E. floccosum* or *M. canis*. Often ring shaped.

Tinea cruris (jock itch)- pink to brown scaling and pruritic plaques involving the groin and thigh but rarely the scrotum or penis, caused by *Tricophyton rubrum*, *T. mentagrophytes*, or *E. floccosum*.

Tinea facialis- dermatophytic erythematous plaque involving the face associated with *T. mentagrophytes, T. ruburm, Maudouinii,* or *M. canis.*

Tinea manuum- scaling and erythematous dermatophyte infection of the hand (usually only one) often associated with tinea pedis, caused by *Tricophyton rubrum, T. mentagrophytes,* or *E. floccosum.*

Tinea pedis (athlete's foot)- scaling and erythematous dermatophyte infection that usually involves the region betweent the fourth and fifth toes but may also involve the lateral and plantar foot, associated with *T. rubrum, E. floccosum, T. mentagrophytes,* and occasionally non-dermatophytes.

Tinea versicolor (Pityriasis versicolor)- asymptomatic localized infection with *P. ovale*; maybe hyper- or hypo- pigmented and scaley.

Tophi - deposits of uric acid in tissues surrounding joints; characteristic of gout.

Toxic epidermal necrolysis- mucocutaneous syndrome associated with prodrome of sore-throat, fever, and headache. In contrast to EM, painful blistering and diffuse sloughing occurs.

Toxic shock syndrome- *S. aureus* exotoxin-mediated pruritic maculopapular eruption characterized by fever, multiorgan failure, desquamation spreading from the hands, associated with tampons or cotton packing.

Trichoepithelioma- benign tumor resembling basal cell carcinoma, characterized by hair differentiation.

Tricholemmoma- squamoid tumor demonstrating basement membrane thickening, epidermal connections, and peripheral palisades.

Trichilemmal cyst (pilar cyst)- scalp nodules composed of a stratified squamous epithelial wall and palisading outer layer, there is no inner granular layer, often familial and occurring in multiples.

Tuberous sclerosis- autosomal dominant proliferation of mesodermal and ectodermal cells, characterized by seizures, mental retardation, hypomelanotic macules, erythematous papules on face, skin-colored plaques, ungual fibromas.

Tylosis- hyperkeratosis of palmar and plantar surfaces.

Ulcer- characterized by loss of the epidermis and papillary dermis, see erosion.

Urticaria- general term to describe any one of a number of conditions that results in generalized wheals, may be acute or chronic. Transient vascular reaction within superficial dermis that results in pruritic localized dermal edema due to dilation and increased permeability of capillaries. There are various causes, most common is allergenic. Angioedema is similar but occurs in deep dermis.

Urticaria pigmentosa- type of macrocytosis characterized by pink to brown plaques which develop a wheal when rubbed (Darier's sign).

Vagabond's disease- eczematization following intense itching with pediculosis corporis (body lice).

Varicella zoster (chicken pox)- contagious *Herpes* virus infection characterized by varying stages of vesicles and crusts.

Varicose veins- enlarged superficial veins due to incompetent venous valves.

Variegate porphyria- combination of findings seen in both porphyria cutanea tarda and acute intermittent porphyria.

Vesicle - fluid filled cystic structure <0.5 cm.

Verrucae vulgaris (common warts)- cutaneous HPV characterized by skin-colored round vegetative papules usually occurring on the hands.

Verrucae plana (flat warts)- pink to violaceous plaques often located on dorsum of hands and feet and caused by HPV.

Verrucae plantaris (plantar warts)- painful hyperkeratotic plaques located on the plantar surface of foot and caused by HPV.

Violaceous - characterized by a violet color.

Vitiligo- white macules; total absence of melanocytes; autoimmune process.

Von Recklinghausen's disease- Neurofibromatosis I.

Weeping - exudation of fluid.

Wegener's granulomatosis- multisystem vasculitis classically involving respiratory tract and kidneys, up to 45% develop a cutaneous vasculitis.

Wen- see epidermoid cyst.

Wheal (hive)- a pruritic pink to red polymorphous plaque occurring secondary to a cutaneous immune response, which is usually transient. See urticaria.

Whipple's disease- Infection cause by *Tropheryma whippelii* affecting nearly every organ system characterized by diarrhea, weight loss, arthropathies, and skin hyperpigmentation in a sun-exposed regions in approximately 45% of cases.

White dermatographism- blanching of the skin in atopic persons in response to stroking with a blunt object, see dermatographism.

Wickham's striae- white, reticular pattern on the surface of lichen planus lesions.

Wrinkle - loss of elastic recoil of skin usually due to a degeneration of elastin fibers but can also be due to over growth of elastin fibers.

Xanthelasma- soft yellow to orange papules on the eyelids occasionally associated with hyperlipoproteinemia.

Xanthoma- yellow to brown papule, plaque, or tendon infiltration, may indicate hyperlipoproteinemia or lymphoma.

Xerosis- pruritic, dry, scaling patch; generalized dry itchy skin.

7

DERMATOLOGICAL SIGNS AND ASSOCIATIONS

Adenoma sebaceum/angiofibromas- tuberous sclerosis.

Acanthosis nigricans- gastric and lung cancer, obesity, polycystic ovary disease, diabetes mellitus, Cushing's disease, acromegaly.

Acrodermatitis- zinc deficiency.

Allergic rhinitis- atopic dermatitis.

Angiokeratomas- Fabry's Disease.

Apple-jelly diascopy- sarcoidosis.

Ash-leaf spots- tuberous sclerosis.

Auspitz's sign- plaques of psoriasis reveal bleeding points when scale removed. Not specific for psoriasis.

Bacillary angiomatosis- primarily in AIDS.

Basal cell epitheliomas- basal cell nevus syndrome.

Beau's lines- period of stress or illness.

Blue nails- minocycline, antimalarials, Wilson's disease, silver-nitrate, ochronosis.

Brown nails- arsenic toxicity, gold, Addison's disease, hemochromatosis, malignant melanoma. See Hutchinson's sign.

Bullae- *tense*- bullous pemphigoid; *flaccid*- pemphigus vulgaris.

Buttonhole sign- invagination with compression by the tip of an index finger, characteristic for neurofibroma.

Calciphylaxis- end-stage renal disease, hyperparathyroidism.

Café au lait spots- neurofibromatosis, Albright's syndrome

Carney complex- LAMB and NAME syndromes.

Champagne bottle sign- inverted champagne bottle shape in lipodermatosclerosis.

Clubbed fingers- cardiac disease, pulmonary disease, colitis, enteritis, hepatic cirrhosis, heritable.

Darier's sign- development of a wheal when a lesion is rubbed.

Dennie-Morgan folds- atopic dermatitis.

Dermatitis herpetiformis- gluten sensitivity, malabsorption.

Dermatographism- urticaria.

Dyshidrotic eczema- atopic dermatitis, contact dermatitis, hyperhidrosis.

Gluteal pinking- psoriasis.

Glucagonoma syndrome- alpha cell tumor of the pancreas.

Gottron's papules/sign- dermatomyositis.

Green nails- pseudomonas infection (usually associated with Candida).

Hand desquamation- TSS, Streptococcus infections, Kawasaki disease.

Hutchinson's sign- proximal nail fold hyperpigmentation in a caucasian suggestive of malignant melanoma.

Hyperlinear palms- atopic dermatitis.

Id reaction- contact dermatitis, stasis dermatitis.

Janeway lesions-infective endocarditis.

Koebner's phenomena- psoriasis, sarcoidosis, lichen planus.

Koilonychia- iron deficiency (esp. Plummer-Vinson syndrome), hemochromatosis, trauma, Raynaud's syndrome, or heritable (Autosomal dominant).

Lichen planus- hepatitis C.

Linear dermatitis- contact dermatitis, esp. to Rhus dermatitis (poison ivy).

Muehrcke's nails- hypoalbuminemia.

Myxedema- generalized=hypothyroidism, pretibial=Grave's disease.

Nail telangiectasia- CTD, dermatomyositis, lupus erythematosus, scleroderma.

Necrobiosis lipoidica- diabetes mellitus.

Neurofibromas- von Recklinghausen's disease.

Neuromas- multiple endocrine neoplasia syndrome, type 2b.

Nikolsky's sign- pemphigus vulgaris and SSSS.

Nocturnal pruritus-scabies.

Onycholysis- hyperthyroidism, trauma, onychomycosis, chemicals, psoriasis.

Osler's nodes- infective endocarditis.

Palm pain-erythema multiforme.

Periungual fibroma- tuberous sclerosis.

Plummer's nails- Grave's disease.

Pressure ulcers- bony prominences.

PUPPP (Pruritc Utricarial Papules and Plaques of Pregnancy)- 3rd trimester, usually primigravidae.

Pyoderma gangrenosum- inflammatory bowel disease (esp. ulcerative colitis).

Satellite papules/pustules- candidiasis.

Sebaceous adenomas- Torre's syndrome.

Shagreen patches- tuberous sclerosis.

Splinter hemorrhages- trauma, infective endocarditis.

Terry's nails- classically hepatic cirrhosis, also congestive heart failure, uremia, or hypoalbuminemia.

Tricholemmomas- Cowden's disease, breast and thyroid cancer.

Toxic Shock Syndrome- tampons, gauze packing.

Venous ulcers- medial leg and malleolus.

White dermatographism- atopic dermatitis.

8

TREATMENTS

ACNE
Although lipophilic bacteria cause acne, removal of oil with astringentsor vigorous washing may exacerbate the condition. Wash face once or twice a day at most.

COMEDONES
Apply one of the following keratolytic agents qhs:
0.1% Adapalene gel,
Tretinoin (begin at low strength of 0.025% cream and increase up to 0.1%),
2% Azelaic acid cream.

MILD INFLAMMATORY PAPULES/PUSTULES
Topical antimicrobial agents ± keratolytics- 5% benzoyl peroxide gel qAM.
Use washes for larger areas such as the back.
Reduce to 2.5% if irritating or increase to 10% if tolerated.
Topical 1% Clindamycin lotion, or 2% Erythromycin ointment (dry skin),
    pledgets, gel, or alcohol-based solution (oily skin).
Sodium sulfacetamide 10% and sulfur 5% lotion
    (antibacterial and antipityrosporum),
    5-8% Sulfur and 2% Recorcinol (keratolytic).
Oral Tetracycline or Erythromycin in doses ranging from 250 – 1000mg/day
    decreases bacterial colonization, has an unknown anti-inflammatory effect.

MODERATE INFLAMMATORY PAPULES/PUSTULES
Topicals as above, and systemic antibiotics for 1-3 mos: Tetracycline 500 mg bid;
Doxycycline 100 mg bid, Erythromycin 250 mg qid, or Minocycline 100 mg qd.

SEVERE NONDULOCYSTIC ACNE OR SCARRING
The synthetic Retinoid isotretinoin 0.5-2.0 mg/kg daily for 3-6 months.

ACNE ROSACEA
Avoid precipitants: spicy food, alcohol, emotional stimuli, hot drinks,
    and other substances that cause vasodilation.
Oral Tetracycline 500 mg qd-bid or 100 mg Doxycycline qd-bid.
Topical Metronidazole (0.075% gel/cream/lotion bid), Novacet and Sulfacet qd.
Ocular disease does not respond to topical agents.
Rhinophyma- electrosurgery or laser.

ACTINIC KERATOSIS
Few lesions- Cryotherapy, Curettage, Electrodesiccation.
Diffuse or numerous-
  5-Florouracil cream 5% or lotion 2% or 5% qd-bid for 3(face)-6(arms) weeks.

ALOPECIA AREATA
Intralesional injection of 2.5-5 mg/ml Triamcinolone acetonide suspension
  (or other dilute corticosteroids) not exceeding 20 mg. Inject q 3-4 weeks.
High potency topical corticosteroid ointments or creams may be used for several
  months with frequent evaluations for atrophy.
Minoxidil and Anthralin have also been used.

ANDROGENIC ALOPECIA
Men:
2-5% topical Minoxidil solution bid
1 mg po Finasteride qd
Women:
2% topical Minoxidil bid

ATOPIC DERMATITIS/ECZEMA/OTHER DRY SKIN DISORDERS
Avoid irritants.
Warm (not hot) baths with bath oil.
Apply lubrication (cream or ointment) immediately after bath.
Mild to mid-potency topical emollient cream or ointment based corticosteroids.
Avoid soap.
Antihistamines for pruritus (first generation/sedating).
Secondary infection-
  Oral antistaphylococcal agents such as Erythromycin 250 mg tid
  or cephalexin 250 mg tid for 7-10 days.
  Burrow's solution (1:40 tid) for weepy lesions.
0.03-0.1% tacrolimus ointment bid is a newer, very promising therapy.
Systemic corticosteroids (30 mg prednisone for 10 days)- only for severe flares.
Refer to allergist for testing if recalcitrant disease and if allergy is suspected.

BASAL CELL CARCINOMA
Cryotherapy, curettage ± electrodesiccation, excision.
Moh's micrographic surgery may be the treatment of choice for ears and central
  face lesions, sclerosing, recurrent, or aggressive lesions.
If surgery cannot be tolerated- radiation therapy.

BULLOUS PEMPHIGOID
Oral Tetracycline 500 mg tid and oral Niacinamide 500 mg tid
  may work for mild cases
Oral prednisone 1-2 mg/kg qd
Methotrexate, Cyclosporine, azathioprine

CALLUSES
Salicylic acid (over-the-counter medication)

CUTANEOUS CANDIDIASIS
Topical Azoles or Nystatin applied twice daily for 2-3 weeks
Systemic Azoles

CONTACT DERMATITIS
Remove or avoid allergen
High potency topical glucocorticoid
Oral corticosteroids (40-60 mg/day; 10-15 days) if severe or on genitalia or face
Contact dermatitis typically lasts 1-3 weeks
If unresponsive to treatment, consider continued exposure to allergen
Perform patch testing if allergen suspected

DERMATOMYOSITIS
Avoid sun and use daily sunscreens
Oral Prednisone 0.5-1 mg/kg qd
If no response, try Oral Methotrexate 15-30 mg q week
    (or Cyclosporine, chlorambucil, azathioprine, cyclophosphamide)
For recalcitrant skin disease- Oral Hydroxychloroquine 200-400 mg qd

DERMATOPHYTOSIS
Topical Azoles or Allylamines for minor lesions:
QD Imidazoles:
    1% Econazole (Spectazole), 1% Oxiconazole (Oxistat), 2% Ketoconazole (Nizoral)
BID Imidazoles: 1% Clotrimazole, 2% Miconazole.
QD Allylamines: 1% Naftifine (Naftin).
BID Allylamine: 1% Terbinafine (Lamisil).
For severe or extensive lesions- Terbinafine 250 mg for 3-4 weeks
Tinea capitis-
    Oral Microsize Griseofulvin 15-22 mg/kg qd
    or Ultramicrosize 10-15 mg/kg for >6 weeks or
    Terbinafine 62.5mg/d (<20kg), 125 mg/d (20-40kg), 250 mg/d (>40kg)

DRUG REACTIONS
Phenytoin hypersensitivity reaction-
    Systemic corticosteroids (0.5 –1.0 mg/kg prednisone),
    Oral antihistamine for pruritus,
    d/c phenytoin, avoid carbamazepine and phenobarbital, which may cross-react.
Photosensitivity- avoid sun.
Pustular eruptions- Resolve rapidly with drug withdrawal
Urticaria-
    drug withdrawal,
    oral antihistamines,
    epinephrine if cardiac or respiratory compromise occurs.
Warfarin necrosis-
    Vitamin K, heparin, protein C replacement if deficient .

DYSPLASTIC NEVUS SYNDROME
Photograph and measure lesions; with follow up every 6-12 months.
Avoid sun and teach ABCD's of malignant melanoma.
Excise worrisome or changing lesions.

EPIDERMOID CYST/EPIDERMAL INCLUSION CYST
If symptomatic or troublesome-
Inject with <0.5 ml intralesional triamcinolone 2.5 – 5.0 mg/ml.
If infection is a concern-
Treat with Erythromycin or Cephalexin 250 mg qid x 7-10d.
Incise and drain if a pustular head is visible ("pointing") for immediate relief.
When inflammation has subsided-
Carefully remove entire cyst wall without spilling contents if possible.

ERYTHEMA MIGRANS
Oral Doxycycline, Tetracycline, Penicillin G, Cefuroxime, Cefotaxime,
Ceftriaxone, or Amoxicillin (in children less than 8 years),

ERYTHEMA MULTIFORME
Eliminate offending agent/medication/infection.
Mild cases are usually not treated.
Fluid replacement and topical antibiotics to prevent secondary bacterial infections.
Oral Prednisone, 1 mg/kg qd x1-3 weeks, for early EM may be beneficial
but use later in the course is controversial.
Oral Acyclovir 200-400mg bid has been used to suppress herpes simplex virus
in herpes-associated EM

FURUNCLE
Incise and drain.
Cephalexin 250-500 mg po tid for 14 days.
Dicloxacillin 250-500 mg po tid for 10 days.
Recurrent lesions:
Treat with Bacitracin or Mupirocin ointment bid.

GRANULOMA ANNULARE
Super-potent topical Glucocorticoid ointments/creams,
Iintralesional steroids,
Cryotherapy.
Lesions usually spontaneously resolve within 6-24 months
Biopsy has been reported to cause lesions to disappear.

HERPES SIMPLEX (HSV)
Acute (primary or recurrent)-
Acyclovir 200 mg PO 5qd for 10d.
Valacyclovir 1000 mg PO bid.
or Famciclovir 125 mg PO bid.
Mucocutaneous HSV-
Acyclovir 200-400 mg PO 5x per day for 10d for immunocompromised.
Intermittent suppressive therapy for genital herpes-
Acyclovir 200 mg PO q 4h (or 5qd) for 5d.
Chronic suppressive therapy for genital herpes-
Acyclovir 400 mg PO bid for up to 1 year.

HERPES ZOSTER
Immunocompetent- usually self-limited.
   To reduce acute neuritis, use
      Oral Acyclovir 800 mg PO q4h (5qd) x7-10d,
      Valacyclovir 1000 mg PO tid x10d,
      or Famciclovir 500 mg PO tid x7d.
   Oral Prednisone 60 mg qd x7d tapered to 30 mg the following week.
      It is controversial whether this is helpful for postherpetic neuralgia.
Immunosuppressed-
   IV acyclovir 500mg/m2 or 10mg.kg q8h x 7-10d.
Disseminated- 5-10 mg/kg IV q8h x7-10d.

IMPETIGO/ECTHYMA
Debridement of crusts with soaks.
Topical antibiotics such as mupirocin ointment 2% tid alone
   or with oral antibiotics.
Oral anti-staphylococcal antibiotics-
   Cephalexin 250 mg tid,
   Dicloxacillin 250 mg tid,
   or Erythromycin 250 mg qid x7-10d.

KERATOCANTHOMA
Excision is the generally accepted treatment
   due to similarities between keratoacanthomas and SCC.

KERATOSIS PILARIS
Avoid irritants, drying, and scratching.
Lubricate aggressively.
12% Lactic acid lotion/cream bid
   or Retin-A (topical tretinoin cream).

LICHEN PLANUS
Usually idiopathic but other etiologies include medication reaction and hepatitis C.
High to super-potent Topical Glucocorticoid creams/ointments.
Recalcitrant or severe cutaneous lesions-
   Dapsone or Retinoids have been tried.
Mucous membranes-(less likely than cutaneous lesions to resolve spontaneously)
   0.5 ml 2-10 mg/ml Intralesional Triamcinolone (max 15 mg per week).

LUPUS ERYTHEMATOSUS
Avoid sun and use sunscreen lotions daily.
Discoid Lesions
   Topical Corticosteroids
   or Intralesional Triamcinolone 0.5 ml or 3mg/ml.
Hydroxychloroquine 200-400 mg qd
   or Chloroquine Phosphate 250-500 mg qd
Severe cases may require cytotoxic agents such as
   Methotrexate, Azathioprine, or Cyclophosphamide.

MILIUM
Use a #11 scalpel blade to incise the lesion.
Express contents with squeezing or a comedone extractor.

MOLLUSCUM CONTAGIOSUM
Curettage, Cryotherapy, Electrodesiccation, laser ablation.

ONYCHOMYCOSIS (Tinea unguium)
Terbinafine 250 mg qd for 6 weeks (fingernails) or 12 weeks (toenails)
Check LFTs approximately 6 weeks after initiation of therapy.

PARONYCHIA (bacterial)
Acute severe paronychia-
     If pustule is visible, use a No. 11 blade to incise and drain.
Treat with cephalexin 250-500 mg qid x7d.

PARONYCHIA (chronic/candidal)
Avoid water contact; Trim nail short
Treat with
     Topical Clotrimazole Solution and equal parts
          10% Na Sulamyd Ophthalmic Solution (sodium sulfacetamide) in 95% ETOH
          bid for 3-6 months
     or Imidazole cream bid or tid,
     or 4% Thymol in Chloroform bid to tid
Recalcitrant or severe-
     add Oral Itraconazole 100-200 mg qd x7d
     or Terbinafine 250 mg for 2-4 weeks to the above regimen.

PEMPHIGUS VULGARIS- see treatment of Bullous pemphigoid.

PEDICULOSIS CAPITIS
1% Lindane or Permethrin shampoo for 10 minutes.
     (Over the counter preparations such as Nix)
Use a Nit Comb with or without white vinegar.
Wash all recently worn clothes in hot water, dry clean, or discard.
Topical corticosteroid creams or ointments are useful for severe pruritus.

PERIORAL DERMATITIS
Low-potency Topical Corticosteroid cream/ointment
     with 1-3% precipitated sulfur, 0.075% Metronidazole cream/gel,
5% benzoyl peroxide, or oral tetracycline 500-1000 mg per day.
Other topical agents that have been used include
     2% Topical Clindamycin and 2% Topical Erythromycin lotion/gel.

PITYRIASIS ROSEA
May last up to 12 weeks.
Low to mid-potency Topical Corticosteroid ointment/cream,
0.25 – 0.5% Phenol or Menthol containing lotions or creams,
Occasionally UV-B phototherapy or sunlight.
Associated Pruritus may be controlled with Antihistamines.

PRURITUS

Rule out underlying disease and treat.

Emollients.

Medium-potency Topical Corticosteroid ointment/cream for local inflammations

0.25 – 0.5% Phenol or Menthol containing lotions or steroid cream/ointments

Oral Antihistamines-

  Cyproheptadine 4 mg, or doxepin 25 – 50 mg, or hydroxyzine 10-25 mg
  at night or up to 4 times per day.

High to super-potent Topical Corticosteroids for

  Prurigo Nodularis or Lichen Simplex Chronicus.

PSEUDO-FOLLICULITIS BARBAE (shaving bumps)

Avoid close shaving and when possible, grow a beard.

Avoid comedogenic lotions, wash with mild soap.

Mild cases-

  Topical antibiotics

    (2% Mupirocin Ointment or Cleocin T/1% Clindamycin lotion).

  5% Benzoyl Peroxide wash bid.

For Itching:

  1% Hydrocortisone cream or ointment.

Diffuse or severe cases-

  Oral antibiotics

    Tetracycline 500 mg bid, 100 - 400 mg

    Doxycycline tid to qid,

    Erythromycin 250 mg qid,

For secondary infection

  Cephalexin.

PSORIASIS

Aggressive lubrication of skin.

Plaque-

  Mid-potency Topical Corticosteroids (tachyphylaxis occurs)

    if <20% body surface

  Consider keratolytic gel, or tar, or Wilson's Wonder (1oz).

  Topical Calcipotriene (vitamin D) ointment/cream/solution 0.005% bid

  or topical Tazarotene gel 0.05% to 0.1% qd.

Older regimens include

  Goeckerman regimen

    (1-5% crude Coal Tar in an ointment base with UV-B light therapy)

  Ingram regimen

    (Anthralin and UV-B).

PUVA- Topical/Oral Psoralens with UV-A, especially if >20% body surface involved.

Scalp-

  Anti-psoriatic/seborrheic shampoo,

  Calcipotriene solution,

  and mid-high potency Topical Steroid solutions.

  Consider keratolytics and sulfur (eg. 1-2-3 cream, please see compounds).

Psoriatic arthritis-

  Methotrexate, Acitretin, and/or Cyclosporine,

  consider referral to a rheumatologist.

RHUS DERMATITIS (Poison Ivy, Oak, Sumac)
1% Hydrocortisone topical cream for up to one week.
Beware of potential for secondary bacterial infections.

SCABIES
5% Permethrin cream or 1% Lindane lotion from head to toe for 12 hours.
Ivermectin 200 ug/kg for severe crusted scabies or recalcitrant cases.
Med to high-potency Topical Corticosteroid cream for severe pruritus.
   Note that pruritus can persist for up to 2 weeks following successful therapy.

SEBORRHEIC DERMATITIS
Low-potency Topical Corticosteroid ointments/creams for face. Shampoos with
Coal Tar and/or Salicylic Acid, Zinc, Sulfur; 2% Ketoconazole shampoo.
Mid-high potency Topical Corticosteroid solutions for scalp.

SEBORRHEIC KERATOSIS
Cryotherapy or curettage if lesions are symptomatic or unsightly.

SKIN TAGS
Cut at base with scalpel or scissors, cryosurgery, electrodesiccation.

SQUAMOUS CELL CARCINOMA
Excision with primary closure and margin evaluation by a dermatopathologist
or Mohs' micrographic surgery in high risk lesions and locations.

STASIS DERMATITIS
Leg elevation to control chronic edema and prevent ulcerations.
Apply 20-40 mmHg compression stockings for ambulation.
Oral antibiotics if severe: (Erythromycin or Cephalexin 250 mg qid for 7-10 days).
Medium to high potency Topical Corticosteroid cream can be used for up to
   several months to reduce inflammation.
Ulcers- gently debride and cover with wound dressing and an Unna boot.

STEVENS-JOHNSON SYNDROME (SJS)
Fluid replacement and topical antibiotics to prevent secondary bacterial infections.
IV Methylprednisolone (2mg/kg qd during the initial 24–72 h) is controversial.
Antihistamines for pruritus.
Groups II-V Topical Corticosteroids for plaques and papules.
Viscous Xylocaine rinse is helpful for symptomatic relief of oral lesions.
Aggressive wound care in a burn unit for extensively denuded skin.

THRUSH
Oral Nystatin suspension 100,000 U/ml tid
or Mycelex (clotrimazole) troches 10 mg dissolved slowly 5x per day for 14 days.

TINEA VERSICOLOR
Selenium Sulfide shampoo 2.5% for 10 minutes qd x10d.
Topical Azoles bid x2wks– prescribe 5-10 g/day depending on area to be covered.
Oral Terbinafine 250 mg qd x7d.
Maintenance is mandatory to prevent recurrence (eg. 1-2 treatments per month).

TOXIC EPIDERMAL NECROLYSIS   See SJS above.
Additional treatments that have been employed:
  Cyclophosphamide (100-300mg IV for 5d) or Cyclosporine.
  Plasmapheresis
  IVIG 0.75 g/kg qd x5d.
  Hyperbaric Oxygen.

UTRICARIA
Antihistamines
Oral Prednisone 1 mg/kg qd for 7 days, alternate course if possible.

VARACELLA ZOATER/SHINGLES
Within 24-72h of rash onset,
  give 10-20 mg/kg PO qid x5d. (max: 800 mg/dose)
  or 10 mg/kg IV q8h x7d.

WARTS
Cryotherapy.
Salicylic Acid with or without Lactic Acid.
Trichloracetic Acid.
Cantharidin.
Electrodesiccation and Curettage.
Carbon Dioxide Laser/Pulse Dye Laser.
Apply 15-25% Podophyllin in Tincture of Benzoin to wart for 2 hours,
  may repeat weekly.
Note most warts spontaneously resolve within 2 years.

APPENDIX A:
TOPICAL STEROIDS ACCORDING TO POTENCY

<u>NOTE</u>: Potency ranges from super potent (group I) to weak (group VII).
<u>Super potent</u>: for palms, soles, chronic, hyperkeratotic, or lichenified lesions.
<u>Low to medium potent</u>: for infants, face, genitalia, intertriginous, or thin lesions.
<u>Base</u>: (O) = ointment (C) = cream (E) = emollient cream (G) = gel (L) = lotion

GROUP I (should not be used for more than 3 weeks)

Generic Name	Brand Name	Sizes (grams)
Aug. betamethasone dipropionate	Diprolene (O)	15, 50
Clobetasol propionate	Temovate (O) 0.05%	15, 30, 45, 60
Clobetasol propionate	Temovate (C) 0.05%	15, 30, 45, 60
Clobetasol propionate	Temovate E (E) 0.05%	15, 30, 60
Diflorasone diacetate	Psorcon (O) 0.05%	15, 30, 60
Halobetasol propionate	Ultravate (O) 0.05%	15, 50
Halobetasol propionate	Ultravate (C) 0.05%	15, 50
Flurandrenolide tape	Cordran tape	24" 80", (12) 2" by 3" patch

GROUP II

Generic Name	Brand Name	Sizes (grams)
Amcinonide	Cyclocort (O) 0.1%	15, 30, 60
Aug. betamethasone dipropionate	Diprolene AF (C)	15, 50
Betamethasone dipropionate	Diprosone (O) 0.05%	15, 45
Desoximetasone	Topicort (G) 0.05%	15, 60
Desoximetasone	Topicort (O) 0.25%	15, 60
Desoximetasone	Topicort (EC) 0.25%	15, 60, 4oz
Diflorasone diacetate	Florone (O) 0.05%	15, 30, 60
Fluocinonide	Lidex 0.05%	15, 30, 60
Fluocinonide	Lidex-E (C) 0.05%	15, 30, 60
Fluocinonide	Lidex (C) 0.05%	15, 30, 60, 120
Fluocinonide	Lidex (G) 0.05%	15, 30, 60
Fluocinonide	Lidex (O) 0.05%	15, 30, 60, 120
Halcinonide	Halog (C) 0.1%	15, 30, 60, 240
Halcinonide	Halog (O) 0.1%	15, 30, 60, 240

GROUP III

Generic Name	Brand Name	Sizes (grams)
Amcinonide	Cyclocort (C) 0.1%	15, 30, 60
Amcinonide	Cyclocort (L) 0.1%	20 ml, 60 ml
Betamethasone dipropionate	Diprosone (C) 0.05%	15, 45
Diflorasone diacetate	Maxiflor (C) 0.05%	30, 60
Mometasone furoate	Elocon (O) 0.1%	15, 45
Fluticasone propionate	Cutivate (O) 0.005%	15, 30, 60
Triamcinolone acetonide	Aristocort A (C) 0.5%	15, 60, 240
Triamcinolone acetonide	Aristocort A (O) 0.5%	15, 60

GROUP IV

Generic Name	Brand Name	Sizes (grams)
Fluocinolone acetonide	Elocon (C) 0.1%	15, 45
Flurandrenolide	Cordran (O) 0.05%	15, 30, 60
Hydrocortisone valerate	Westcort (O) 0.2%	15, 45, 60
Mometasone furoate	Elocon (C) 0.1%	15, 45
Triamcinolone acetonide	Kenalog (O) 0.1%	15, 60, 240

GROUP V

Generic Name	Brand Name	Sizes (grams)
Betamethasone dipropionate	Diprosone (L) 0.05%	60 ml
Fluocinolone acetonide	Synalar (C) 0.025%	15, 60
Flurandrenolide	Cordran (C) 0.05%	15, 30, 60
Flurandrenolide	Cordran (L) 0.05%	15 ml, 60 ml
Hydrocortisone butyrate	Locoid (C) 0.1%	15, 45
Hydrocortisone valerate	Westcort (C) 0.2%	15, 45, 60
Mometasone furoate	Elocon (C) 0.1%	15, 45
Triamcinolone acetonide	Kenalog (C) 0.1%	15, 60, 80
Triamcinolone acetonide	Kenalog (L) 0.1%	60 ml

GROUP VI

Generic Name	Brand Name	Sizes (grams)
Alclometasone dipropionate	Aclovate (C) 0.05%	15, 45, 60
Alclometasone dipropionate	Aclovate (O) 0.05%	15, 45, 60
Desonide	DesOwen (L) 0.05%	2 fl oz, 4 fl oz
Desonide	DesOwen (O) 0.05%	15, 60
Desonide	Tridesilon (C) 0.05%	15, 60, 5 lbs.
Fluocinolone acetonide	Synalar (TS) 0.01%	20 ml, 60 ml

GROUP VII

Generic Name	Brand Name	Sizes (grams)
Hydrocortisone	Hycort (C) 1%	1 oz
Dexamethasone	Decaspray (10mg/25g)	25
Flumethasone	Locarten (C) 0.03%	15

NOTE:

Preparation may be grouped differently depending upon source of information.

Dispensing directions:

Prescribe enough to be used BID for one week
This requires estimating the amount needed based on the patient's surface area.
Approximations for one week supply for the average adult:

Full body	200g
Leg	60g
Chest/Back	45g
Arm/both feet	30g
Face/neck/both hands	15g
Head	15g
Genito-anal	15g

APPENDIX B:

SIDE EFFECTS, INTERACTIONS, CONTRAINDICATIONS OF COMMONLY PRESCRIBED MEDICATIONS

NOTE:
This is not a comprehensive list. Consult medication manufacturer for more details.

Acyclovir-
Acute renal failure (especially if given rapid IV injection), coma, leukopenia, thrombocytopenia, seizures, neuropsychiatric toxicity (esp. immunocompromised and geriatric patients).
Common effects- local phlebitis (parenteral), lethargy, GI disturbances, arthralgias, lightheadedness, headaches, lethargy, confusion.
Contraindicated if hypersensitivity to acyclovir exists.
Caution in impaired renal function or with nephrotoxic drugs.

Adapalene-
Burning, pruritus, erythema, scaling.

Cephalexin-
Severe- neutropenia, thrombocytopenia, anaphylaxis, pseudomembranous colitis, common- diarrhea, nausea, vomiting, headache, dizziness, increased LFTs, eosinophilia.
Contraindicated if hypersensitive to cephalexin.
Caution if allergic to penicillin, history of pseudomembranous colitis, impaired renal function, lactating, using nephrotoxic agents.

Doxycycline-see tetracycline, increased photosensitivity.

Erythromycin-
Abdominal pain, nausea, vomiting, oral candidiasis, cholestatic jaundice, rare ventricular arrhythmias, fever, hypertrophic pyloric stenosis, rash, fever, diarrhea, pseudomembranous colitis, eosinophilia, cholestatic jaundice, other.
Contraindicated.

Finasteride-
Decreased libido, decreased ejaculate, impotence, other.
Contraindicated if hypersensitive to finasteride, female.

5-Florouracil-
Severe inflammation (as expected), photosensitivity, other.
Contraindicated if hypersensitive, pregnancy, lactation.
Caution with impaired hepatic function.

Griseofulvin-
Urticaria, rash, headache, fatigue, insomnia, confusion, photosensitivity, nausea, vomiting, abdominal pain, diarrhea, oral thrush, rare- angioneurotic edema, GI bleeding, menstrual toxicity, hepatic toxicity, proteinuria, leukopenia, nephrosis,

other.
Contraindicated if hypersensitive to griseofulvin or penicillin, severe liver disease, porphyria.
Caution in children <2yo, long-term therapy, pregnancy, avoid excess sunlight exposure.

Isotretinoin- Accutane-
Oral prescription medication approved by the FDA for the treatment of severe recalcitrant nodular acne. It is a known human teratogen that can cause major embryopathies associated with maternal exposure. Some of which include cranio-facial, cardiac, thymic, and central nervous system malformations. It is imperative to avoid pregnancy during exposure and a pregnancy.

Minocycline- see tetracycline,
Dizziness (and other CNS toxicity), blue pigmentation of skin and mucous membranes. May be taken with food or milk.
Contraindications- see tetracycline, caution not needed in renal impairment.

Minoxidil solution- pruritus, erythema, contact dermatitis.
Contraindicated if hypersensitive to minoxidil or pregnant.
Caution in pts with hypertension, other cardiovascular disease, and >50yo (no information available for this population).

Prednisone and other corticosteroids-
Adrenal insufficiency, psychosis, peptic ulcers, CHF, anaphylaxis, Long term, severe- osteoporosis, immunosuppression, Peds- pseudotumor cerebri, pancreatitis, common- dyspepsia, nausea, vomiting, edema, increased appetite, headache, euphoria, irritability/anxiety, insomnia, hypokalemia, hyperglycemia, hyperten-sion, menstrual irregularities, acne, ecchymosis. Long-term, common: Cushingoid features, skin atrophy, impaired wound healing.

Terbinafine-
Neutropenia, hepatic toxicity or failure, EM, SJS, TEN, anaphylaxis
Common- headache, dyspepsia, abdominal pain, nausea, diarrhea, constipation, flatulence, rash, pruritus, urticaria, elevated LFTs, taste or visual changes,
Contraindications- hypersensitivity to terbinafine, not recommended for pregnancy, not approved for Pediatrics.
Caution with impaired renal or liver function- check LFTs.

Tetracycline-
Neutropenia, thrombocytopenia, hemolytic anemia, hepatotoxicity, pseudotumor cerebri, increased ICP and skeletal growth retardation in infants, tooth discoloration if <8yo, pericarditis, anaphylaxis, pseudomembranous colitis.
Common- dyspepsia, esophagitis, diarrhea, nausea, vomiting, photosensitivity, stomatitis, oral and vaginal candidiasis, phlebitis (parenteral), CNS disorders, tinnitus, elevated BUN.
Contraindicated if hypersensitive to tetracycline or similar medications, pregnancy, <8yo. Caution with impaired renal or hepatic function.

APPENDIX C:
TOPICAL MEDICATION VEHICLES

GEL
Elegant formulation, usually alcohol-based, contains a gelling agent that liquifies on contact with skin. Useful for hair-bearing regions or when drying is desired.

LOTION
Emulsion of oil and water, like cream but less moisturizing and more liquid consistency.

CREAM
Emulsion of oil and water, less moisturizing than ointments but more cosmetically acceptable. Some are **Emollient** (high oil content) and some are **Drying** (little to no oil content). Use for acute and subacute dermatoses. May be used for moist lesions and intertriginous regions.

OINTMENT
Greasy vehicle which provides enhanced penetration. Best choice for dry skin, hyperkeratotic and lichenified lesions. Not to be used on moist lesions. Especially useful for chronic atopic dermatitis.

SOLUTION
A liquid vehicle: propylene glycol, water, or alcohol.
Ideal for use under cosmetics, hair-bearing regions, and when drying is desired.

APPENDIX D:
USEFUL COMPOUNDS

COMPOUND	INGREDIENTS	APPLICATION
Wilson's Wonder	LCD 8% Salicylic acid 4% 0.025% triamcinolone (O)	Eczema, Psoriasis
Greer's Goo	Nystatin powder (1 mill Units/oz.) Hydrocortisone (1% pwdr 300 mg/oz.) Zinc oxide QSAD	Candida intertrigo, Intertriginous psoriasis
1,2,3 Cream	Hydrocortisone 1% (C) Salicylic acid 2% Precipitated sulfur 3%	Seborrheic dermatitis Intertriginous psoriasis

APPENDIX E:

<u>PHOTOGRAPHS</u>:
SELECTED SKIN LESIONS

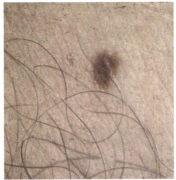

Junctional Nevus: Note the uniform coloration and smooth borders.

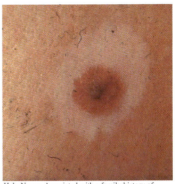

Halo Nevus: Associated with a family history of vitiligo. Eventually, the central nevus may disappear.

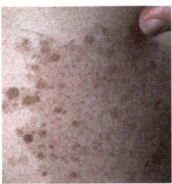

Nevus Spilus: The scattered nevi within this, typically benign, macule may be flat or raised.

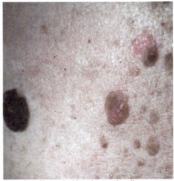

Seborrheic Keratosis: Note the "stuck-on" appearance and various coloration patterns of these papilliform papules-nodules. Closer examination reveals plugged follicles or "horny cysts."

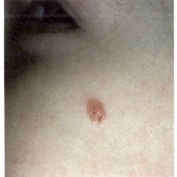

Spitz Nevus: This well-circumscribed dome-shaped nodule on the cheek of this child developed rapidly over several months.

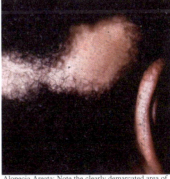

Alopecia Areata: Note the clearly demarcated area of alopecia characterized by non-erythematous, smooth, non-scaling skin.

65

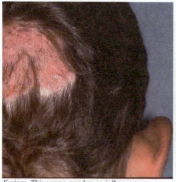

Kerion: This young man has an inflammatory, edematous crusted plaque that may scar upon healing, it is a reaction to a dermatophyte infection.

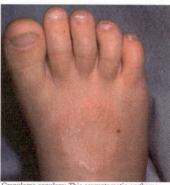

Granuloma annulare: This asymptomatic erythematous annular plaque is often found on the hands, feet, and extensor surfaces of arms and legs.

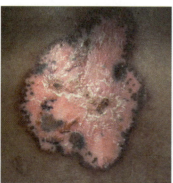

Discoid Lupus Erythematosus: An erythematous well-demarcated plaque wtih central atrophy.

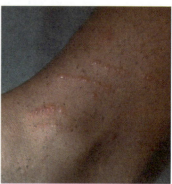

Rhus Dermatitis (Poison Ivy Dermatitis): Note the linear arrangement of this delayed cell-mediated reaction to a plant.

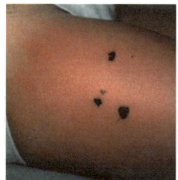

Rhus Dermatitis (Poison Ivy Dermatitis): Indurated erythematous lesions still contain black lacquer-like oxidized resin from the poison ivy plant. Sometimes misdiagnosed as spider bite.

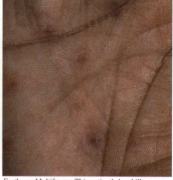

Erythema Multiforme: This patient's hand illustrates the typical "target" lesions and their initial distal presentation.

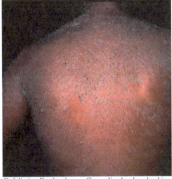

Exfoliative Erythroderma: Generalized red scaly skin.

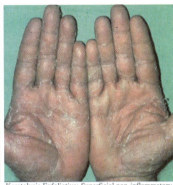

Keratolysis Exfoliativa: Superficial non-inflammatory peeling of palmar and/or plantar skin.

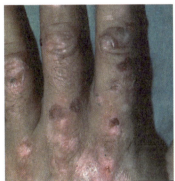

Porphyria Cutanea Tarda: Note vesicles, crusts, scars caused by minor trauma. Hypertrichosis of the face and scleroderma-like changes on sun-exposed skin may occur as well.

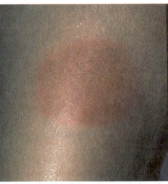

Fixed Drug Reaction: Solitary plaque on the leg will likely recur in the same location if re-challenged by same offending drug. Lesion resolves within weeks after the drug withdrawn.

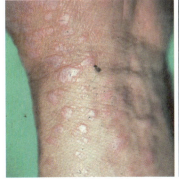

Lichenoid Drug Eruption: Note the violaceous shiny papules and plaques.

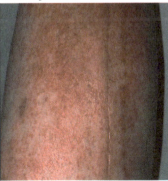

Thiazide Capillaritis: Note the typical cheyenne-pepper-like macules seen on the legs of this patient following treatment with HCTZ.

67

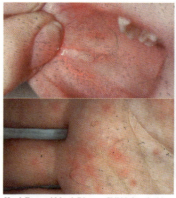

Hand, Foot and Mouth Disease: Child infected with Coxackie A16. Minimal symptoms, highly contagious

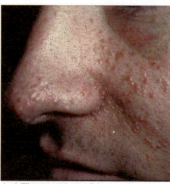

AngioFibromata (Adenoma Sebaceum): Dome-shaped erythematous papules pathognomic for Tuberous Sclerosis.

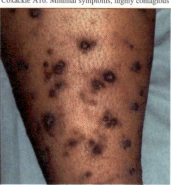

Prurigo Nodularis: Discrete, firm, intensity pruritic nodules caused by chronic scratching or rubbing.

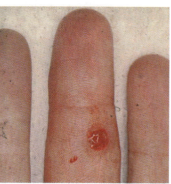

Pyogenic Granuloma: Aka Lobular Capillary Hemangioma. Red bleeding hemangioma develops rapidly from minor trauma. Particularly common during pregnancy.

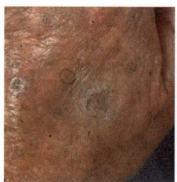

Actinic Keratosis (Solar Keratosis): Erythematous lesions with adherent scale; sometimes tender.

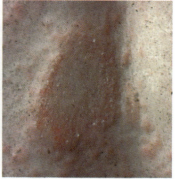

Pityriasis Rosea: This herald patch developed approx 1-2 weeks prior to a generalized eruption that has a "Christmas tree" distribution on the trunk.

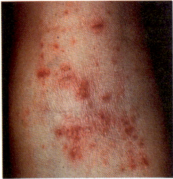

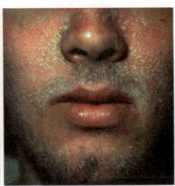

Atopic Dermatitis: Eczema, "The itch that rashes," is characterized by numerous excoriations as seen on the flexor surface of this arm.

seborrheic Dermatitis: Erythema and scaling typically occur in regions with numerous sebaceous glands, eye brows, scalp, behind the ears. "Cradle Cap" in infants.

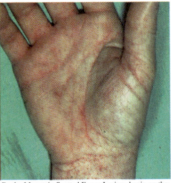

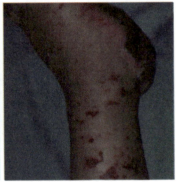

Rocky Mountain Spotted Fever: Lesions begin on the wrists and ankles; spread to palms, soles and trunk. Erythematous and blanchable, then petichial. Season April to Sept. With fever, myalgia, and headache.

Meningococcemia (Purpura Fulminans): Stellate purpura is typical for fulminant N.menigitis infection with DIC (Disseminated Intravascular coagilation).

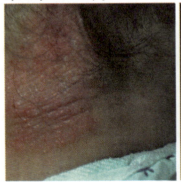

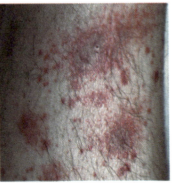

Lichen Simplex Chronicus: This patient had chronic pruritus from atopic dermatitis and often rubbed her neck. Such lichenified plaques are also common on legs, thighs, extensor forearms, and pubic region.

Palpable Purpura: Non-blanchable, hemorrhagic papules are typical for Cutaneous Vasculitis.

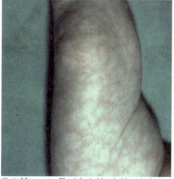

Cutis Marmorata: Physiologic blanchable reticular rash due to immature cutaneous neurovasculature. Also seen in women in cold environment.

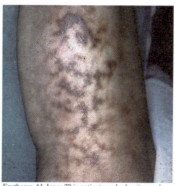

Erythema Ab Igne: This patient used a heating pad frequently and developed this brownish reticular erythematous lesion.

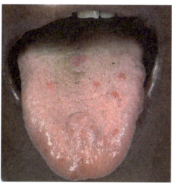

Hereditary Hemorrhagic Telangiectasia (Osler-Weber-Rendu): Punctate and papular telangiectasias of mucus membranes, fingers, and palms appear post-puberty in this patient with epistaxis and family history of HHT.

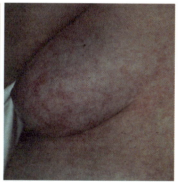

Poikiloderma Vasculare Atrophicans: Hyper and hypo pigmented telangiectasias with atrophy are present in PVA - seen in patients with MF or diabetes mellitus.

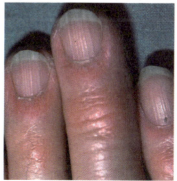

Dermatomyositis: Periungal telangiectasia, erythema due to dilated and infarcted capillary loops; also seen SLE and, rarely, in progressive systemic sclerosis.

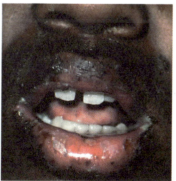

Stevens-Johnson Syndrome: This patient has painful mucosal erosions. Some patients develop eruptions indistinguishable from TEN.

70

MELANOMA

<u>Defintition</u>- Malignant tumor that arises from the melanocytic system of the skin or other organs which contain melanocytes.
(see Nevi and other Pigmented Lesions chapter for more details about sub-types of melanoma.

<u>The ABCD's that raise concern for melanoma</u>:

    Asymmetry
    Border irregularities
    Color abnormalities (especially black, and numerous colors within one mole)
    Diameter greater than 6mm (a pencil eraser)

<u>Staging</u>:
I: <1.5cm. II: >1.5cm. III: spread to regional lymph nodes. IV: distant metastases.

<u>Treatment</u>:
Surgical excision with wide margin, and regional lymph node dissection.
Adjuvant therapy with chemotherapy, immunotherapy, and radiation therapy.
Surgical resection of metastatic lesions (brain, viscera), palliative care (incurable if metastatic).

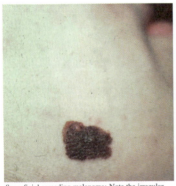

<u>Superficial spreading melanoma</u>: Note the irregular border, black and red coloration of this cheek lesion.

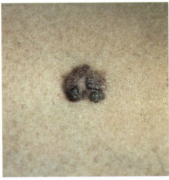

<u>Superficial spreading melanoma with small nodules</u>: Note asymmetry, border irregularities, and abnormal coloration of this lesion that is only 0.6mm.

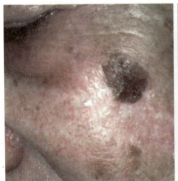

<u>Lentigo maligna melinoma</u>: Typically located on face of elderly patient. This "melanoma in-situ" is usually characterized by slow growth.

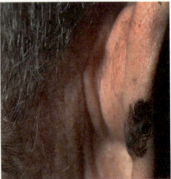

<u>Melanoma on posterior ear</u>: Note this often overlooked location for melanoma.

71

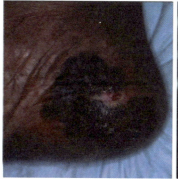
Acral lentiginous melanoma: Occurs mostly in older males of African or Asian descent. Other locations include palms, mouth, anus and genitalia.

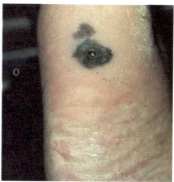
Acral lentiginous melanoma: Occurs mostly in older males of African or Asian descent. Other locations include palms, mouth, anus and genitalia.

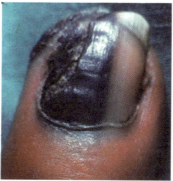
Sub and periungual melanoma: Acral lentiginous melanoma subtype. Note involvement of proximal nailbed and lateral folds (see Hutchinson's sign). May be misdiagnosed as subungual hematoma.

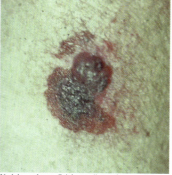
Nodular and superficial spreading melanoma: This nodular lesion developed in a region of superficial spreading melanoma. Evidence of regression worsens the prognosis.

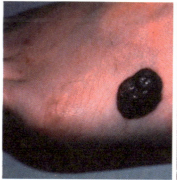
Nodular melanoma: Black multilobulated lesion arose from a congenital nevus on the foot of this patient.

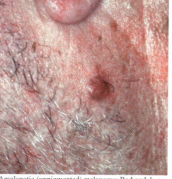
Amelanotic (unpigmented) melanoma: Red nodule on this patient's face could be easily overlooked.